BLOOD TYPE DIET

Eat Right For Your Blood Type

Crystal Moore

this book are for clarifying purposes only and are the owned by the owners themselves, not affiliated with this document.

Table of Content

Introduction..7

Blood Type Diet Pros and Cons...9

Pros...9

Cons..9

Blood Type Diet for Type A..11

Food List for Type A...11

Blood Type Diet for Type B...16

Food List for Type B..16

Blood Type Diet for Type AB...21

Food List for Type AB...21

Blood Type Diet for Type O..26

Food List for Type O..26

Grocery Lists for Blood Type Diet..30

Grocery List for Type A...30

Grocery List for Type B...30

Grocery List for Type AB...31

Grocery List for Type O...32

FAQs..34

Blood Type A Diet Recipes...36

1) Amaranth Crackers..36

2) Vegetable Trio...37

3) Ginger Carrots and Hijiki...38

4) Herbal Cheesy Balls...39

5) Carrot and Honey Soup..40

6).Lentil Patties...41

7) Pineapple Smoothie...42

8) Apricot and Apple Soup...43

9) Spinach and Carrot Wrap..44

10) Kale Crisps...45

Blood Type B Diet Recipes...46

1) Baked Carrot and Apple Casserole...46

2) Baked Fish Pate...47

3) Baked Sweet Potato 48

4) Delicious Beet Greens 49

5) Better Flax Biscuits... 50

6) Blueberry Vanilla–Flavoured Cookies 51

7) Flax Oats Muffins 52

8) Millet Veggie Bread 53

9) Quinoa Muffins 54

10) Soy Oatmeal Cookies (High Protein).. 55

Blood Type AB Diet Recipes 56

1) Potato Tuna Salad.. 56

2) Broccoli Salad... 57

3) Quick Zucchini Salad... 58

4) Pumpkin Salad 59

5) Spelt and Flax Bread 60

6) Spinach and Yogurt Dip 61

7) Tofu Egg Salad 62

8) Walnut Apple Muffins.. 63

9) Gluten-Free Flax and Millet Crackers 64

10) Lemony Shortbread Bars 65

11) Lemon and Poppy seed Muffins 66

Blood Type O Diet Recipes 67

1) Sweet and Sour Fish 67

2) Artichoke and Spinach Dip 69

3) Simple Japanese Salmon... 70

4) Smoky Beef-Brisket 71

5) BBQ Meatballs 72

6) Almond Flax muffins.. 73

7) Amaranth and Quinoa Gingerbread Muffins 74

8) Blueberry and Buckwheat Bread.. 75

9) Carrot Muffins 76

10) Gingerbread 77

11) Gluten-Free Cinnamon-Flavoured Flax-Cranberry Muffins 78

12) Gluten-Free Ginger Cinnamon Cookies 80

13) Nut and Honey Almond Slices 81

14) Banana Oat and Buckwheat Bread 82

15) One-Bowl Cupcakes...83

16) Cherry and Parsnip Bread 84

17) Pineapple and Walnut Cookies...85

18) Pumpkin Vanilla–Flavoured Muffins 86

19) Fast Savoury Bread...87

Introduction

The lack of correct nutrition has resulted in the development of several unique approaches for healthy eating. Amongst them, the Blood Type Diet has emerged as an intriguing nutritional plan.

The Blood Type Diet was developed by Dr. Peter J. D'Adamo, the author of the book *Eat Right for Your Type*. According to Dr.D'Adamo, the strength of the diet lies in the fact that it gives a personalized approach to eating for each blood group. This diet is proven to be an extremely popular diet used by a lot of people to prevent or remedy diseases, lose weight, and maintain an ideal weight. This diet is also called BTD or ER4YT (the acronym of his book).

According to the theory behind *"Eat Right for Your Type"* by Peter J D'Adamo, a chemical reaction takes place between our blood and the foods that we eat. This reaction is a part of our genetic inheritance and is caused by the diverse and abundant proteins found in foods called lectins. These proteins contain agglutinating (clumping) properties that affect our blood, so when we eat a food that contains lectins that are incompatible with our blood type antigen, these lectins target a bodily system or an organ and start to agglutinate the blood cells in that region. The Blood Type Diet is designed to target these types of specific factors.

According to Dr.D'Adamo, our blood type may determine which illnesses and diseases we may develop. It is an interesting approach, however, no research has been conducted, and no studies have been conducted that show blood type may be a predictor for development of certain kinds of diseases.

Considering what was said before, the basic principle of this diet is, not everybody should follow the same diet—our blood type and race will determine the tolerance to what we should and shouldn't eat. Based on this principle, there are sixteen food groups that are neutral, highly beneficial, or detrimental. Each blood type is supposed to eat in the following way:

- **Type A:** Called cultivator, or agrarian. Type A people should eat a plant-based diet that is totally free of toxic red meat. This very much resembles a vegetarian diet.

- **Type B:** Called nomad. Type B people can eat most meats (except pork, duck, goose, hens and chicken) and plants, and they can eat some dairy. However, they must avoid corn, wheat, tomatoes, lentils, all shellfish, eel, snail, ice cream, American cheese and blue cheese.

- **Type AB:** Called enigma. It is a combination between Types A and B. Foods to eat include tofu, dairy, seafood, grains, and beans. They have to avoid kidney beans, beef, corn, and chicken.

- **Type O:** Called hunter. This high-protein diet is based mainly on fish, meat, poultry, and certain vegetables and fruits, but it limits legumes, grains, and dairy. This resembles the paleo diet.

Blood Type Diet Pros and Cons

Pros

Lots of people have in fact reported good results with the Blood Type Diet. However, as with many other famous eating plans, there are some people who question the nutritional advantages of this diet and the lack of scientific evidence supporting Dr.D'Adamo's claims. Aside from this, the opinion that blood type affects almost every aspect of an individual's health is widely accepted.

Moreover, any increases in exercise or healthy changes in eating are going to benefit an individual's health, and all changes that Dr.D'Adamo suggests in every plan can possibly result in weight loss. Although an individual's success from this plan may be more attributed to a lifestyle change, you will still see the beneficial effects of eating based on your blood type.

The strength of the Blood Type Diet is that it encourages people to find a personalized diet that suits their digestive system and to increase their level of physical activity. Overall, the recommendations for most of the blood types are good. Also, the Blood Type Diet, by helping people reduce their calorie intake, can lead to weight loss. Unlike many other fad diets, the general advice of this diet is sound.

Cons

Medical experts universally say that there is absolutely no link between our blood group and the diet we eat. Consequently, this diet is not recommended by qualified dieticians or nutritionists. There are also a number of concerns that the diets prescribed for blood groups A and O are significantly limited, and they cut out a majority of food groups. In the long term, this may result in an insufficient intake of nutrients that are required for good health. Eliminating dairy products, for example, leads to an insufficient intake of calcium, which in turn can put us at a risk for osteoporosis (brittle bone disease), while avoiding animal protein (meat) may result in low intake of iron, which in turn can lead to anaemia.

Another concern is that the diet for type O is too protein-heavy. Animal protein, particularly red meat, is linked to health problems like colorectal cancer and heart disease.

While this diet may help with weight loss, whether it has more considerable health benefits is a different matter entirely. Critics of this diet say that there is little to no science to back up its theory that eating per blood type may improve our health. There is no single well-designed study that either confirms or refutes the benefits of the Eat Right for Your Type diet.

Blood Type Diet for Type A

Blood type A people have more sensitive digestive systems than the other blood types, and for them, D'Adamo prescribes a basically vegetarian diet. According to him, Type A people should avoid dairy foods and meat and should focus on fruits, vegetables, and whole grains.

Type A people are predisposed to cancer, heart disease, and diabetes. It is especially important for sensitive Type A people to get as natural food as possible—pure, fresh, and organic. When we follow a Type A Diet, we will be thinner naturally. We will supercharge our immune system and potentially prevent the development of life-threatening diseases.

Food List for Type A

Meats and Poultry

Type A people should limit the quantity of meat consumed.

Most Beneficial: None

Foods Allowed: Chicken, turkey, Cornish hens

Foods Not Allowed: Pork, beef, veal, venison, goose, and duck

Seafood

Most Beneficial: Cod, carp, grouper, monkfish, red snapper, salmon, sardine, white fish, pickerel, rainbow trout, sliver perch, sea trout, snail, and yellow perch

Foods Allowed: All kinds except those listed as not allowed

Foods Not Allowed: Anchovy, barracuda, bluefish, beluga, bluegill bass, clam, caviar, catfish, crab, conch, crayfish, eel, frog, flounder, grey sole, hake, haddock, halibut, herring, lox, lobster, mussels, oysters, octopus, shad, scallop, shrimp, squid, sole, striped bass, turtle, and tilefish

Dairy

Most dairy products are not digestible for Type A people.

Most Beneficial: None

Foods Allowed: Yogurt, feta, mozzarella, ricotta, goat cheese, string cheese, goat milk, and kefir

Foods Not Allowed: Milk and all other cheeses

Fats

Most Beneficial: Olive oil, flaxseed oil

Foods Allowed: Cod liver oil, canola oil

Foods Not Allowed: Oil of cottonseed, peanut, corn, sesame and safflower

Nuts

Most Beneficial: Peanuts, pumpkin seeds

Foods Allowed: All kinds except those listed as not allowed

Foods Not Allowed: Brazil nuts, cashews, pistachios

Beans

Type As flourish on vegetable proteins found in legumes and beans.

Most Beneficial: A duke, black, azuki, pinto, green, red soy, black-eyed peas, lentils

Foods Allowed: All types except those listed as not allowed

Foods Not Allowed: Copper, kidney, garbanzo, Lima, red, navy, and tamarind (these beans may cause a decrease in production of insulin for Type As)

Grains

Type As normally do well on grains and cereals. They should select more concentrated whole grains in place of instant, processed cereals.

Most Beneficial: Amaranth, buckwheat

Foods Allowed: None

Foods Not Allowed: Cream of wheat, farina, familiar, grape nuts, granola, seven grain, wheat germ, shredded wheat, durum wheat, wheat bran

Bread and Noodles

Type As have wonderful options in pastas and grains.

Most Beneficial: Bread (Essene, Ezekiel, sprouted wheat, soya flour), rice cakes, flour (rice, oat, rye), pasta (artichoke), soba noodles

Foods Allowed: All types except those listed as not allowed

Foods Not Allowed: Bread (multi-grain, high-protein, whole wheat), English muffins, wheat bran muffins, matzos, pumpernickel, flour (whole wheat, white), pasta (spinach, semolina)

Vegetables

Vegetables are very important to the Type A diet, and they provide enzymes, minerals, and antioxidants. Type As should eat vegetables in a state as natural as possible (steamed or raw) in order to preserve their complete benefits.

Most Beneficial: Garlic, onions, carrots, broccoli, collard greens, kale, spinach, pumpkin (These vegetables boost immune systems of Type As.); artichoke, chicory, horseradish, greens (Swiss chard, dandelion), romaine, okra, leek, parsley, alfalfa tempeh, sprouts, tofu, turnip

Foods Allowed: All types except those listed as not allowed

Foods Not Allowed: Peppers, potatoes, olives, yams, sweet potatoes, cabbage, tomatoes, eggplant, lima beans, and mushrooms (Type A people are extremely sensitive to these vegetables. These have a strong, harmful effect on the Type A digestive tract.)

Fruits

Most fruits are allowed for Type As, although giving more emphasis to alkaline fruits may help to balance grains, which are acid forming in Type As' muscle tissues.

Most Beneficial: Berries (blueberries, blackberries, cranberries, boysenberries), plums, figs, prunes; pineapples, apricots, cherries (The digestive enzyme in these fruits is a great digestive aid for Type As.); lemon, grapefruit (These fruits show alkaline tendencies after digestion, which has a positive effect on Type As' stomachs.)

Foods Allowed: All types except those listed as not allowed

Foods Not Allowed: Melons, honeydew, cantaloupe, mangoes, bananas, papaya, coconuts, oranges, tangerines, rhubarb

Spices

The right combination of spices may be powerful boosters for the immune systems of Type As.

Most Beneficial: Tamari, soy sauce, miso, garlic, ginger

Foods Allowed: None

Foods Not Allowed: Vinegar, pepper (black, white, and cayenne), plain gelatine, capers, and wintergreen (the acids are likely to cause irritation to the stomach lining)

Condiments

Most Beneficial: None

Foods Allowed: None

Foods Not Allowed: Ketchup, mayonnaise, pickles, relish, Worcestershire sauce (Type A should avoid these products because they have low levels of stomach acid.)

Beverages

Most Beneficial: Hawthorn, aloe, burdock, alfalfa, green tea, Echinacea, red wine (1 glass per day) (These beverages may help to improve immune system for Type As.); slippery elm, ginger, coffee (1 cup per day) (These beverages may help Type A to enhance their stomach-acid secretions.)

Foods Allowed: None

Foods Allowed: Beer, seltzer water, distilled liquor, black tea, soda (These beverages don't suit the digestive systems of Type As, nor do they support their immune systems.)

Blood Type Diet for Type B

Type B People can digest a wide range of foods; however, they should still avoid some foods, as they could contribute to weight gain. These foods include corn, lentils, buckwheat, sesame seeds, and peanuts. They should avoid gluten products but eat red meat, eggs, green vegetables, low-fat dairy foods, oats, liquorice tea, soy, millet, flaxseed, and spelt.

The strong and attentive Type B people are normally able to resist various, and the most severe, diseases common in modern life, like cancer and heart disease. Actually, Type B people who carefully follow the recommended diet may often bypass severe diseases and live a long, healthy life. Type B people are more likely to get immune-system disorders like multiple sclerosis, chronic fatigue syndrome, and lupus.

The diet for Type B is balanced and wholesome, and it includes a wide range of foods. Type B people are the only people who can completely enjoy a wide variety of dairy products.

Food List for Type B

Poultry and Meat

Most Beneficial: Lamb, rabbit, mutton, venison (These meats can help to boost the immune system.)

Foods Allowed: Beef, pheasant, veal, turkey

Foods Not Allowed: Chicken, duck, goose, Cornish hens, quail, pork, and partridge (These meats have a Type B blood agglutinating leptin.)

Seafood

White fish and deep-ocean fish are excellent for Type B.

Most Beneficial: Cod, salmon, halibut, sole, flounder, trout

Foods Allowed: All types except those listed as not allowed

Foods Not Allowed: All shellfish (crab, lobster, mussels, shrimp, crayfish, clam, oysters, etc.), anchovy, beluga, barracuda, eel, lox, octopus, frog, sea bass, striped bass, snail, turtle, yellowtail (These sea foods are badly digested by Type B people. They are disruptive to the Type B system.)

Dairy

Type B is the only blood type that can fully enjoy a variety of dairy foods. That's because the primary sugar in the Type B antigen is D-galactosamine, the very same sugar present in milk.

Most Beneficial: Cottage cheese, feta, farmer, goat cheese and milk, mozzarella, ricotta, kefir, milk, yogurt

Foods Allowed: All types except those listed as not allowed

Foods Not Allowed: American cheese, blue cheese, string cheese, ice cream

Fats

Most Beneficial: Olive oil

Foods Allowed: None

Foods Not Allowed: Canola, cottonseed, peanut, corn, safflower, sunflower, sesame (These oils are not allowed as they contain lectins that can cause damage to Type B digestive tract)

Nuts

Most nuts and seeds are not recommended for Type B people. They contain lectins that interfere with insulin production for Type B people.

Most Beneficial: None

Foods Allowed: All types except those listed as not allowed

Foods Not Allowed: Cashews, pine, pistachio, filberts, peanuts, pumpkin seeds, sunflower seeds, sesame seeds

Beans

Lentils, black-eyed peas, garbanzos, Beans (pintos, azuki, a duke, black) (These beans may interfere with insulin production for Type B people)

Grains

Wheat reduces insulin efficiency and fails to stimulate fat burning in Type B people.

Most Beneficial: Millet, puffed rice, rice (flour, bran), oatmeal (flour, bran), spelt

Food Allowed: All types except those listed as not allowed

Food Not Allowed: Wheat (bran, durum, germ bulgur, white, whole), cream of wheat, shredded wheat, or any products like flour, noodles, and bread made with these grain products; rye and any products like flour, noodles and bread made with these grain products (Rye contains a lectins which settles in vascular system resulting in blood disorder and potentially strokes.); buckwheat, corn (cornmeal, cornflakes) and any products like flour, noodles, and bread made with these grain products (They contribute to sluggish metabolism, fluid retention, insulin irregularity, and fatigue.)

Breads

Most Beneficial: Brown rice, Ezekiel, essence, wasa, fin crisp, rice cakes, millet

Food Allowed: All types except those listed as not allowed

Food Not Allowed: Bagels, bread (whole wheat, multi-grain rye), muffins (bran, corn), soba noodles, couscous, and wild rice

Vegetables

Most Beneficial: Green leafy vegetables (They contain magnesium, an important antiviral agent that helps Type B people fight off autoimmune diseases and viruses.)

Food Allowed: All kinds except those listed as not allowed

Food Not Allowed: Tomatoes (These contain lectins that irritate the stomach lining for Type B people.); corn (This has metabolism- and insulin-upsetting lectins for Type B people.); olive (The mold in it may trigger allergic reactions.); artichoke, avocado, olives, corn, pumpkin, radishes, tempeh, tofu, sprouts

Fruits

Most Beneficial: Pineapples (They have enzymes that help Type B people to digest food more easily.); bananas, grapes, cranberries, papaya, plums

Food Allowed: All types except those listed as not allowed

Food Not Allowed: Coconuts, pomegranates, prickly pear, persimmons, rhubarb, and star fruit

Spices

Most Beneficial: Ginger, curry, horseradish, cayenne pepper (Type B people do best with warming herbs)

Food Allowed: All types except those listed as not allowed

Food Not Allowed: Barley malt sweeteners, Cornstarch, corn syrup, cinnamon (Sweet herbs are likely to be stomach irritants for Type B people.); allspice, gelatine, almond extract, pepper (white and black)

Condiments

Most Beneficial: None

Food Allowed: None

Food Not Allowed: Ketchup

Beverages

Generally, Type B people don't get overwhelming benefits from many herbal teas.

Most Beneficial: Ginger, peppermint, rose hips, raspberry leaf, sage, green teas; ginseng (This is greatly recommended for Type B people as it seems to have a positive effect on their nervous system.); liquorice (It has some antiviral properties.)

Food Allowed: None

Food Not Allowed: Aloe, corn silk, coltsfoot, fenugreek, goldenseal, gentian, hops, mullein, linden, red clover, senna, rhubarb, skullcap, shepherd's purse, distilled liquor, soda, and seltzer water

Blood Type Diet for Type AB

Blood Type AB people can eat a mix of Type A and B diets. The blood type AB is rare, and Type AB people should avoid most of the foods that are listed for Type A and B. Tomato is an exception, and Type AB people can tolerate them. In general, tofu, dairy foods, seafood, green vegetables, Spirulina, pineapple, and sea kelp are foods that Type AB people should include, and beans, red meat, seeds, corn, wheat, and buckwheat should be avoided.

Multiple antigens make Type AB people similar to Type As by having weak stomach acids, and similar to Type Bs by being genetically planned for consumption of meat. Type AB people can't metabolize meats efficiently due to low stomach acid; hence, it is essential to watch portion sizes and frequency. Chicken contains a lectin that irritates the digestive tracts and blood of Type AB people. Tofu is a great protein supplement. Nuts, seeds, legumes, and beans present a mixed picture for Type AB people. Eat seeds and nuts in small quantities and with a little caution.

Type AB people can tolerate dairy products fairly well, but they should watch out for excess mucus production. Generally, Type AB people do well on grains. Type AB people benefit from a diet rich in rice. They have weaker immune systems, so they will benefit from vegetables, which are rich in phytochemicals, and more alkaline fruits, which may help for balancing the grains that are acid forming in muscle tissues. Tomatoes do not impose any ill effect on Type AB people.

Food List for Type AB

Poultry and Meat

Type AB people don't produce sufficient stomach acid for effectively digesting excessive animal protein. The key is to watch portion sizes and frequency. Cured meats may cause stomach cancer for Type AB people with low levels of stomach acid.

Most Beneficial: Lamb, mutton, turkey, rabbit

Food Allowed: All types except those listed as not allowed

Food Not Allowed: Beef, chicken, duck, goose, Cornish hens, partridge, veal, pork, venison, and quail

Seafood

People with a family history of breast cancer should introduce snails (Helix pomatia) into their diet.

Most Beneficial: Tuna, grouper, cod, hake, mackerel, monkfish, mahi-mahi, ocean perch, porgy, trout, pike, red snapper, pickerel, sardine, sailfish, snail, shad, sturgeon

Food Allowed: All types except those listed as not allowed

Food Not Allowed: All shellfish (crab, lobster, mussels, shrimp, crayfish, clam, oysters, etc), anchovy, beluga, bluegill bass, barracuda, flounder, halibut, herring, haddock, eel, lox, frog, octopus, striped bass, sea bass, turtle, and yellowtail

Diary

Soured and cultured products are easily digested for Type AB people.

Most Beneficial: Yogurt, non-fat sour cream, kefir, egg, goat cheese and milk, mozzarella, ricotta

Food Allowed: All types except those listed as not allowed

Food Not Allowed: Blue cheese, American cheese, buttermilk, brie, ice cream, parmesan, camembert, provolone, whole milk, sherbet

Fats

Use sparingly

Most Beneficial: Olive oil

Food Allowed: None

Food Not Allowed: Cottonseed oil, corn oil, sesame oil, safflower oil, sunflower oil

Nuts

Type AB people are likely to suffer from gallbladder problems; hence, nut-butters are preferable over whole nuts. Also, eat small quantities with caution.

Most Beneficial: Walnuts, peanuts (powerful immune boosters for Type AB)

Food Allowed: All types except those listed as not allowed

Food Not Allowed: Filberts, pumpkin seeds, sesame seeds, poppy seeds, and sunflower seeds

Beans

Most Beneficial: Lentils (These beans are an important cancer-fighting food for Type AB. They contain cancer-fighting antioxidants.); pinto, navy, red, soy

Food Allowed: All types except those listed as not allowed

Food Not Allowed: Azuki, aduke, garbanzo, black, fava, black-eyed peas

Grains

The inner kernel of wheat grain is greatly acid forming for Type AB people. Wheat is not recommended if Type AB people are trying to lose weight. Type AB people benefit from a diet rich in rice instead of pasta.

Most Beneficial: Millet, oatmeal, oat bran, puffed rice, rye, rice bran, spelt, and sprouted wheat, and any products like flour, noodles and bread made with these grain products; all types of rice and any products like flour, noodles, and bread made with these

Food Allowed: All types except those listed as not allowed

Food Not Allowed: Corn, buckwheat (any products like flour, noodles and bread made with these), Kamut, soba noodles, kasha, and artichoke pasta

Vegetables

Fresh vegetables are an important source of phytochemicals that have a tonic effect in prevention of heart disease and cancer, diseases that affect Type AB people more often because of their weaker immune systems.

Most Beneficial: Broccoli, cauliflower, beets, celery, green leafy vegetables, eggplant, garlic, cucumber, Maitake mushroom, parsnips, sweet potatoes, parsley, alfalfa sprouts, tofu, tempeh, all kinds of yams

Food Allowed: All types except those listed as not allowed

Food Not Allowed: Artichoke, all type of corns, avocado, black olives, lima beans, all types of bell peppers, Mung bean sprouts, radishes, radish sprouts

Fruits

Emphasize more alkaline fruits for balancing the grains which are acid forming in muscle tissues for Type AB. Fruits rich in vitamin C may help prevent stomach cancer because of vitamin C's antioxidant properties.

Most Beneficial: All types of plums and grapes, berries (gooseberries, cranberries, loganberries), cherries, pineapples (Most tropical fruits do not agree with Type AB, however, pineapple is a great digestive aid.); grapefruits, lemons (Grapefruit exhibits alkaline tendencies after digestion, and lemons help with digestion and clearing mucus from the system); kiwi

Food Allowed: All types except those listed as not allowed

Food Not Allowed: mangoes, guava, bananas, coconuts, oranges (Oranges are stomach irritants for Type AB people; they also interfere with absorption of essential minerals.)

Spices

Kelp and sea salt should be used instead of table salt. Kelp has immensely positive benefits for immune system and heart.

Most Beneficial: Kelp, curry, miso, garlic (a natural antibiotic and potent tonic for Type AB people), parsley, horseradish

Food Allowed: All types except those listed as not allowed

Food Not Allowed: Allspice, anise, almond extract, capers, barley malt, Cornstarch, corn syrup, tapioca, gelatine; vinegar, pepper (black, white, cayenne, red flakes) (These **Ingredients** are acidic.)

Beverages

Most Beneficial: alfalfa, chamomile, Echinacea, burdock, green tea (Type AB people employ these herbal teas for rev up their immune system); liquorice, hawthorn, red wine (1 glass per day) (These beverages and herbal teas build protection against cancer and cardiovascular disease.); dandelion, strawberry leaf, burdock root (These herbal teas may help in the absorption of iron and prevent anaemia.); coffee or decaf coffee (1 cup per day) and alternate day use of green tea (Coffee increases stomach acid and contains the same enzymes found in soy.)

Food Allowed: None

Food Not Allowed: Distilled liquor, black tea, sodas

Blood Type Diet for Type O

The most common blood type is Type O, and Dr.D'Adamo claims that Type O people are more likely to face metabolic issues and weight gain than other types of blood. Blood type O people should eat a low-carb and high-protein diet. Foods recommended for Type O people for weight loss include red meat, seafood, sea kelp, and vegetables, including spinach, kale, and broccoli. Type O people should avoid ham, bacon, some kinds of fish, nuts, grain foods, dairy foods, herbal teas, and coffee. Type O people should not eat specific items including cabbage, avocados, eggplant, mushrooms, corn, olives, oranges, blackberries, melon, coconuts, tangerines, and strawberries.

Type O people flourish on animal protein and intense physical exercise. Unlike other blood types, Type O people's muscle tissue must be slightly on the acidic side. Type O people can efficiently digest and metabolize meats as they are likely to have high content of stomach acid. The success of the Type O diet will depend on use of chemical-free lean meats, fish, and poultry.

Type O people should restrict the use of dairy products because their digestive systems are not designed for proper metabolism.

Food List for Type O

Meat/Protein

The more stressful one's job or demanding one's exercise program, the higher the grade of protein they should eat. Type O people can efficiently digest and metabolize meat. Many seafood are also a great source of iodine that regulates thyroid function.

Most Beneficial: Beef, lamb, veal, mutton, venison, cod, mackerel, herring (Cold-water fish are excellent for Type O people.)

Food Allowed: Any meat or fish except those listed as not allowed

Food Not Allowed: Bacon, ham, pork, goose, barracuda, catfish, pickled herring, caviar, smoked salmon, octopus, and conch

Dairy

Type O people need to restrict the use of dairy food products and eggs

Most Beneficial:

Food Allowed: Butter, feta, mozzarella, farmer, goat cheese, soy milk

Food Not Allowed: All other dairy food products and yogurts

Fat

Type O people respond well to oils.

Most Beneficial: Flaxseed oil, olive oil

Food Allowed: Sesame oil, canola oil

Food Not Allowed: Corn oil, cottonseed oil, peanut oil, safflower oil

Grains

Type O people don't tolerate whole wheat products.

Most Beneficial: Ezekiel bread, Essene bread

Food Allowed: Amaranth, buckwheat, barley, rice, kasha, millet, Kamut, rye, spelt

Food Not Allowed: Corn, graham, gluten, wheat (bulgur, sprouted, durum, white and whole, bran and germ) farina, seven grains, oat, or any products like flour, noodles, and bread made with these grain products

Vegetables

Most Beneficial: Kale, romaine lettuce, broccoli, collard greens, spinach, artichoke, chicory, garlic, horseradish, dandelion, onions, okra, parsnips, parsley, red peppers, pumpkin, seaweed, sweet potatoes, turnips

Food Allowed: Tomatoes; All other types except those listed as not allowed

Food Not Allowed: Brassica family: cabbage, cauliflower, Brussels sprouts, mustard greens (These vegetables inhibit thyroid function for Type O people.); nightshades: potatoes, eggplant; corn, avocado, leek

Fruits

Most Beneficial: Plums, figs, prunes, (Dark red, purple, and blue fruits are likely to cause an alkaline reaction to digestive tract, and thus balance high acidity of Type O people's digestive tract for reducing irritations and ulcers of stomach lining.)

Food Allowed: Grapefruit, most of the berries; all types except those listed as not allowed

Food Not Allowed: Melons, honeydew, cantaloupe, tangerines, oranges, and strawberries, rhubarb, blackberries; coconut and coconut-containing products (Type O people are very sensitive to coconut.)

Spices

Most Beneficial: Kelp-based seasonings, iodized salt (These are rich sources of iodine for regulating the thyroid gland.); parsley, cayenne pepper, curry (soothing to digestive tracts of Type O people)

Food Allowed: None

Food Not Allowed: Black and white pepper, capers, cinnamon, vinegar, Cornstarch, corn syrup, vanilla, nutmeg

Condiments

Most Beneficial: None

Food Not Allowed: Chocolate, cocoa, honey

Food Allowed: Ketchup, mayonnaise, pickles, and relish

Beverages

Most Beneficial: Seltzer water, tea, and club soda

Food Not Allowed: Wine

Food Allowed: Beer, coffee, black tea, distilled liquor

Grocery Lists for Blood Type Diet

Grocery List for Type A

Vegetables:

Garlic, onions, broccoli, carrots, collard greens, kale, pumpkin, spinach, artichokes, chicory, greens, okra, parsley, alfalfa sprouts, tempeh, tofu and turnips.

Fruits:

Berries, plums, prunes, figs, pineapples, cherries, apricots, grapefruit and lemons

Grains:

Amaranth, buckwheat

Seeds:

Peanuts, pumpkin seeds

Oils:

Flaxseed oil, olive oil

Seafood:

Carp, cod, red snapper, rainbow trout, grouper, sardines, salmon, whitefish

Grocery List for Type B

Meats/Proteins:

Lamb (mutton), venison, rabbit

Seafood:

Flounder, grouper, halibut, mahi-mahi, haddock, monkfish, pike, salmon, sea trout, ocean perch, sole, sturgeon and caviar

Dairy:

Feta, cottage, ricotta, goat, mozzarella, yogurt

Oils:

Olive oil

Vegetables:

All leafy green vegetables, beets, Brussels sprouts, cabbage (white, red, Chinese), carrots, cauliflower, eggplant, mushrooms (Shiitake), mustard greens, peppers (green, jalapeno, red, yellow), sweet potatoes, yams

Fruits:

Plums, bananas, grapes (any variety), cranberries, pineapple, papaya

Spices/Herbs:

Curry, cayenne, horseradish

Grocery List for Type AB

Meats/Proteins:

Lamb, mutton, turkey, rabbit

Seafood:

Tuna, grouper, cod, hake, mackerel, monkfish, mahi-mahi, ocean perch, porgy

Dairy:

Yogurt, non-fat sour cream, kefir, egg, goat cheese and milk, mozzarella, ricotta

Oils:

Olive oil

Nuts:

Walnuts, peanuts

Grains:

Millet, oatmeal, oat bran, puffed rice, rye, rice bran, spelt

Vegetables:

Broccoli, cauliflower, beets, celery, green leafy vegetables, eggplant, garlic, cucumber, Maitake mushrooms, parsnips, sweet potatoes, parsley, alfalfa sprouts, tofu, tempeh, all kinds of yams

Fruits:

Plums, grapes, berries (gooseberries, cranberries, loganberries), cherries, pineapples, grapefruits, lemons, kiwi,

Spices/Herbs:

Kelp, curry, miso, garlic, parsley, horseradish

Grocery List for Type O

Meats/Proteins:

Beef, lamb, mutton, veal, venison, Cornish hens, chicken, duck, turkey, eggs

Seafood:

Bluefish, cod, halibut, fresh herring, hake, mackerel, pike, red snapper, salmon, rainbow trout, sardines, shad, sole, striped bass, snapper, sturgeon, swordfish, white perch, whitefish, tilefish, yellow perch, yellowtail

Dairy:

Mozzarella (non-fat), Sour cream (non-fat), eggs, butter, goat cheese, feta cheese, soy cheese, soy milk

Oils/Fats:

Linseed oil, olive oil, canola oil, cod liver oil, sesame oil, almond butter

Nuts/Seeds:

Macadamia nuts, pumpkin seeds, walnuts, chestnuts, pine nuts, sesame seeds, sunflower seeds

Grains:

Amaranth, buckwheat, barley, millet, rice bran, rice, brown rice bread, spelt, quinoa

Vegetables:

Artichoke, Florida avocado, broccoli, broccoli sprouts, beet leaves, chicory, collard greens, escarole, garlic, dandelion, horseradish, kale, kohlrabi, leek, okra, onions, parsley, romaine lettuce, parsnips, red peppers, pumpkin, sweet potatoes.

Fruits:

Kiwi, pineapple, priunes, apples, plums, apricots, bananas, cherries, cranberries, blueberries

Spices/Herbs:

Curry, kelp, cayenne pepper, parsley, Tabasco, turmeric

FAQs

What is a lectin?

A lectin is a protein molecule commonly found in foods that selectively cause our blood and body tissues to agglutinate, or stick together. A lectin that causes tissues of a person with a certain blood type to stick together may not necessarily have the same effect on a person with a different blood type. Lectins also play an important role in hormonal reactions.

How long will we have to be on this diet?

Selecting foods in this manner represents a commitment for a lifetime. It is always up to us to decide which foods we eat. Some people state that they had unfavourable reactions to foods, which they learned to avoid after choosing beneficial options for a six-month period. Others stated that they had a better tolerance for former distressing foods. Only time will tell how we will react.

How do I get started?

There are two ways to get started: 1) For the "cold-turkey "method, quit the foods to avoid and immediately replace them with beneficial foods; 2) the other option is to eat the stocked avoids and then phase them out by replacing them with beneficial foods.

Can a person's blood type change?

Changes in blood type happen only in very rare situations and with certain types of cancers present. The most common cause of changed blood type is antigen sensitivity of chemicals that are used for testing the blood.

I started to lose weight in the first few weeks when I chose to eat food by my blood type, but then I stopped losing weight. What's going on?

The first thing to understand is that selecting foods by blood type is primarily about total health. Weight loss may be a nice side effect of the beneficial food selection. As bodies get healthier, there are various levels one will go through where hormones and glands begin to reset and normalize their duties. During these phases, it is very common not to lose weight.

Patience and 100 percent avoidance of all the foods to avoid is required during this period, which may last one year or more.

How long will it take to see results?

It depends on where you are starting from. Some people start to feel better and show disease remission signs within two weeks. Usually, it takes around two months, and in certain cases, it may be as long as six months for significant results to occur. Weight loss may begin in as little as two weeks or as long as two to six months, depending upon your present glandular state of health.

I appear to be reactive/allergic to an extremely beneficial food. What should I do?

Do not eat it. In the event your body is altered by drugs, disease or surgery, you can have different tolerances for food. In this situation, the best thing to do is avoid allergenic foods and the foods to avoid for your blood type. Choose as many beneficial foods as possible. This sensitivity may perhaps change over time.

Blood Type A Diet Recipes

1) Amaranth Crackers

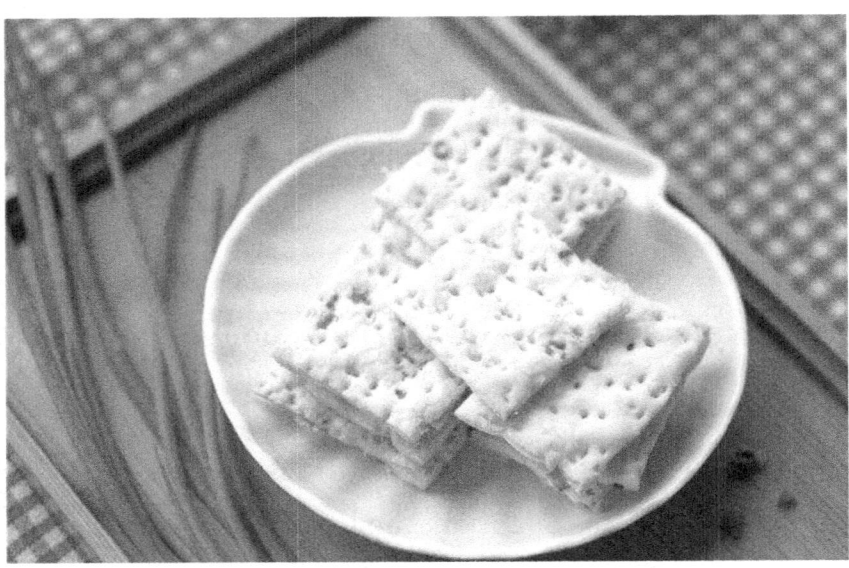

Cooking Time: 8 minutes

Servings: 4

Ingredients:

> ➤ 1 cup of amaranth flour (¼ cup amaranth flour for rolling)
> ➤ 1 tbsp of arrowroot flour
> ➤ 1 tsp of ground dried chives (or any other desired herb)
> ➤ 1 tbsp of flaxseed whole or ground (optional)
> ➤ 2 tbsp of olive oil
> ➤ 2 tsp of sea salt
> ➤ ½ cup of water

Directions:

1. Preheat the oven to 400° F.
2. Mix together the dry Ingredients in a bowl.
3. In another bowl, mix oil and water; beat with fork.
4. Slowly add oil/water to the dry Ingredients, turning the flour slowly.
5. Combine the Ingredients until they form a firm ball.
6. Grease the baking pan and roll out the balls of dough until they are ⅛-inch thick.
7. Place them in the oven for about 3–5 minutes.
8. Remove and flip the crackers, and place them back into the oven for 3 more minutes.
9. Serve them warm or cold.

2) Vegetable Trio

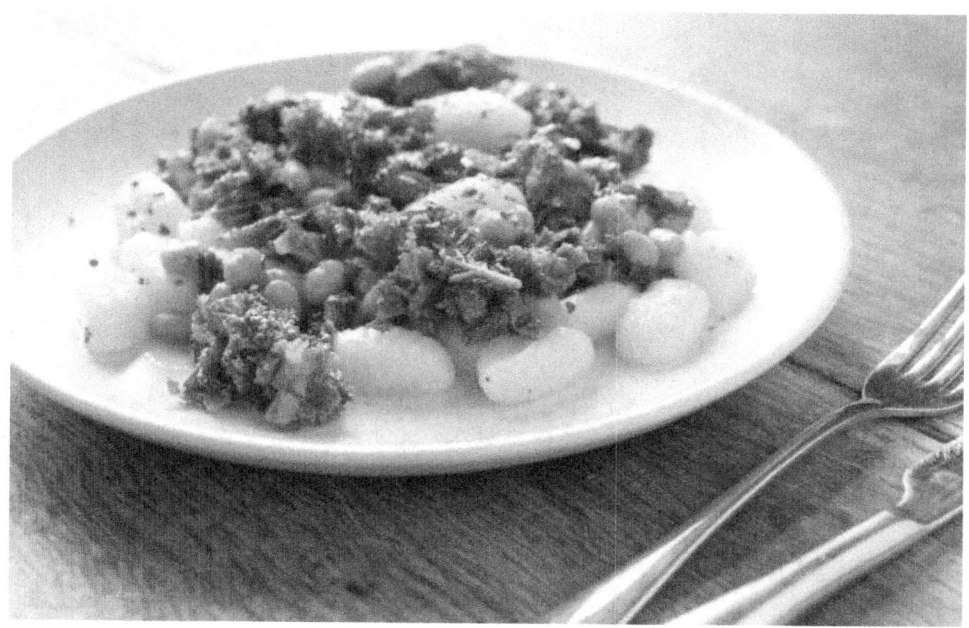

Cooking Time: 23 minutes

Servings: 6

Ingredients:

- 1 large onion
- 1 tsp of grape seed oil
- 1 bunch of fresh kale
- 1 (16 oz) pkg. of frozen black-eyed peas
- salt, to taste

Directions:

1. Chop onion.
2. In a pot, cook onion in oil until it becomes translucent.
3. Add 1 cup of water and black-eyed peas.
4. Bring it to a boil and then reduce the heat; cook for 20 minutes.
5. Separate the kale leaves from stems and tear the leaves into bite-size pieces.
6. Add these to pot.
7. Stir until kale wilts.
8. Cover it and cook until kale becomes tender.
9. Add salt to taste and serve.

3) Ginger Carrots and Hijiki

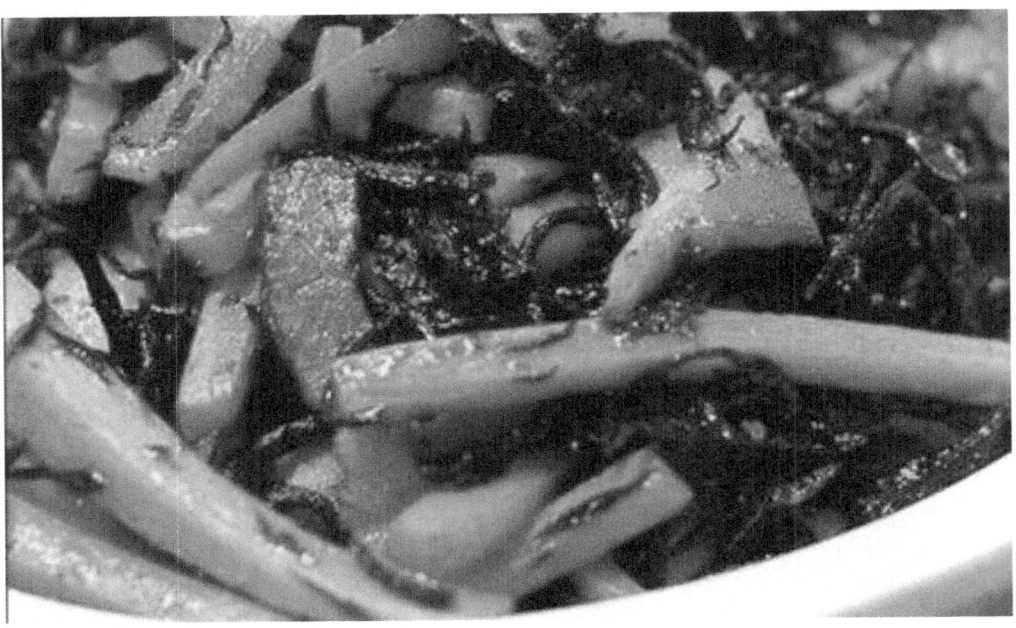

Cooking Time: 30 minutes

Servings: 2

Ingredients:-

- ¼ cup of Hijiki(purchase online), loosely packed
- 1 tsp of extra-virgin olive oil or toasted sesame oil
- 1 tsp of ginger, minced
- 1 clove of garlic, minced
- 1 small carrot, sliced into matchsticks
- 1 small onion, sliced
- 1 tbsp of soy sauce or tamari
- 1 tbsp of mirin (optional)

Directions:

1. Rinse Hijiki; soak it in ½ cup of water for about 10 minutes.
2. Drain and reserve soaking water; chop Hijiki.
3. Warm oil in the skillet, add and sauté onion, ginger, garlic, Hijiki, and carrot for about 5 minutes.
4. Add soaking water and tamari; cover it and simmer for about 15 minutes.
5. At this point, add mirin, if using, adjust seasoning, and serve.

4) Herbal Cheesy Balls

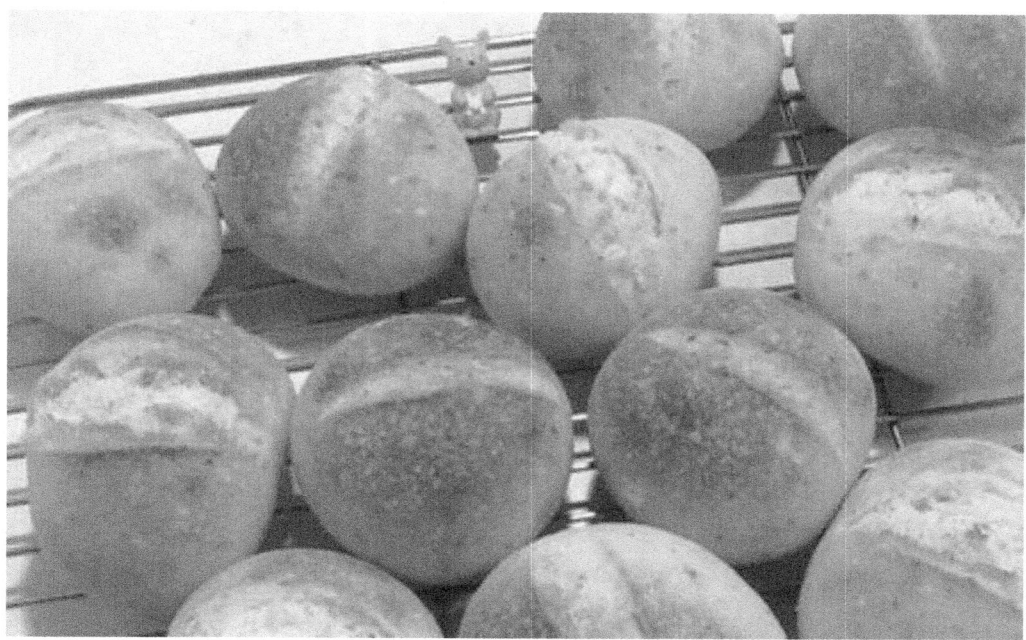

Prep Time: 10 minutes

Servings: 4

Ingredients:

- ➢ 8 oz of cream cheese
- ➢ 1 tbsp of fresh chives, snipped
- ➢ 2 tsp of onions, finely chopped
- ➢ 1 clove of garlic, crushed
- ➢ ½ tsp of dry sage
- ➢ ½ tsp of dry basil
- ➢ ¼ tsp of dry thyme
- ➢ 1 pinch of sea salt
- ➢ 4 drops of hot pepper sauce (if allowed)
- ➢ 3 tbsp of fresh cilantro or parsley, minced

Directions:

1. Combine all the Ingredients except cilantro or parsley.
2. Adjust the seasonings to taste.
3. Shape the mixture into balls.
4. Chill them at least for one day.
5. Remove them 1 hour prior to serving.
6. Roll them in cilantro or parsley and serve them with veggie sticks or rice crackers.

5) Carrot and Honey Soup

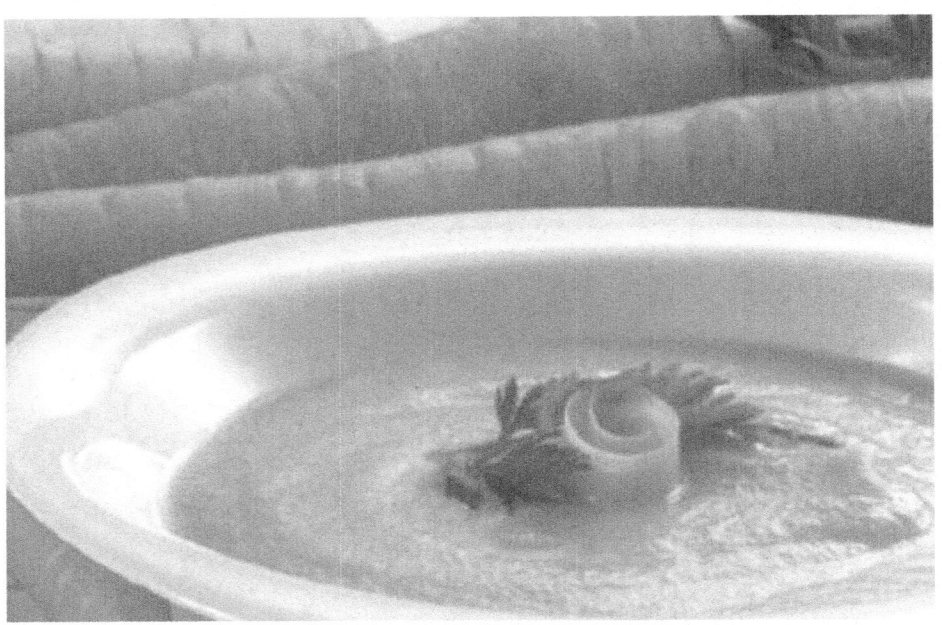

Cooking Time: 30 minutes

Servings: 2

Ingredients:-

> - 1 (16 oz) pkg. of baby carrots
> - 1 cup of vegetable or chicken broth
> - ½ cup of soy milk (or any other milk)
> - ½ cup of honey (or agave syrup)
> - ½ medium onion, chopped
> - ⅛ tsp of nutmeg (to taste)
> - ½ tsp of curry powder (optional)

Directions:

1. Mix carrots, onion, and broth in a saucepan.
2. Cover it; simmer on medium heat for about 15 minutes, or until carrots become tender.
3. Transfer the mixture to a blender and blend until smooth.
4. Return it to saucepan.
5. Add honey and milk and simmer again.
6. Sprinkle it with nutmeg and curry powder and serve it hot or chilled.

6).Lentil Patties

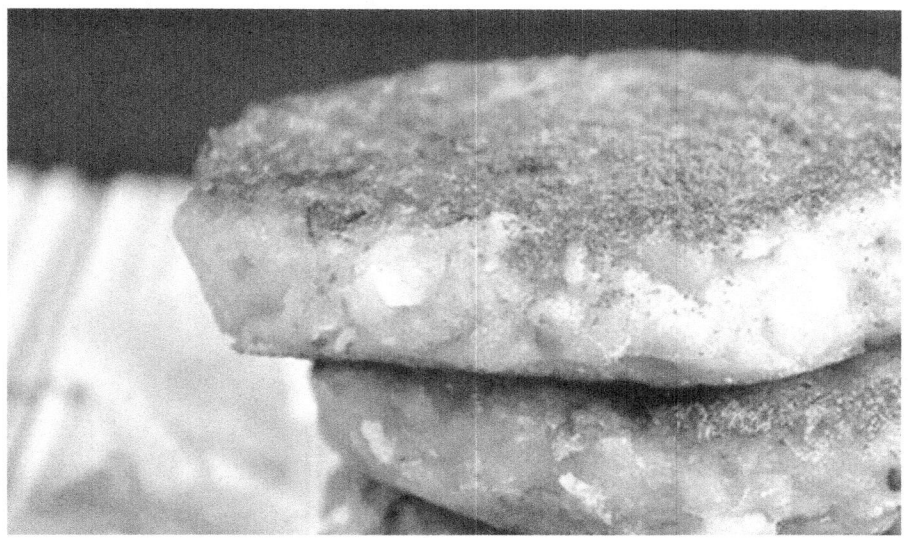

Cooking Time: 15 minutes

Servings: 6

Ingredients:

> - 8 oz of drained lentils
> - 1 egg
> - ½ tsp of sea salt
> - ½ cup of onion, diced
> - 1 tsp of paprika
> - 1 carrot, grated
> - ½ cup of capsicum, diced
> - ½ cup of herbs (parsley, chives, etc.), chopped
> - 2 tbsp of amaranth or rye flour
> - 1 tbsp of olive oil

Directions:

1. Whisk the egg and add remaining Ingredients.
2. Form the mixture into patties.
3. Cook them in olive oil and firmly press down occasionally to get a flat product.
4. Cook until crisp and fairly brown on both sides.

7) Pineapple Smoothie

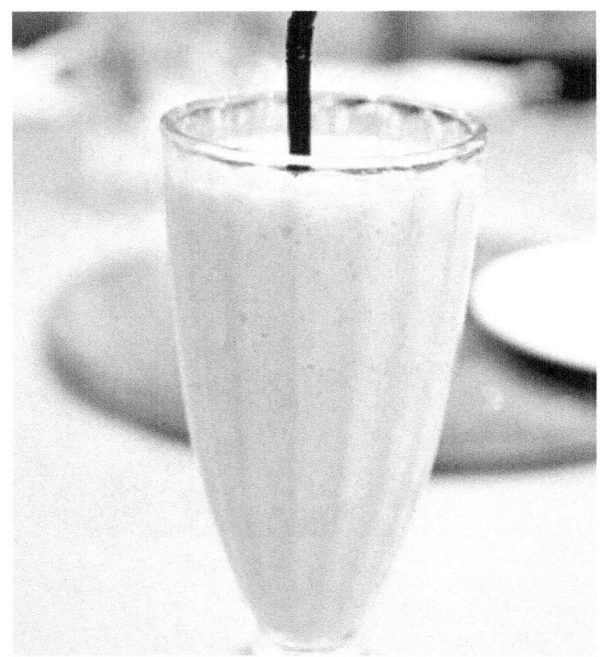

Prep Time: 5 minutes

Servings: 1

Ingredients:

> ➢ 1 cup of Pineapple chunks along with juice
> ➢ 4–5 Strawberries
> ➢ water
> ➢ 1 scoop of soy protein powder
> ➢ a little bit of sugar or maple syrup

Variations: add cinnamon, some cranberries

Directions:

1. Blend all Ingredients in a blender until smooth and serve.

8) Apricot and Apple Soup

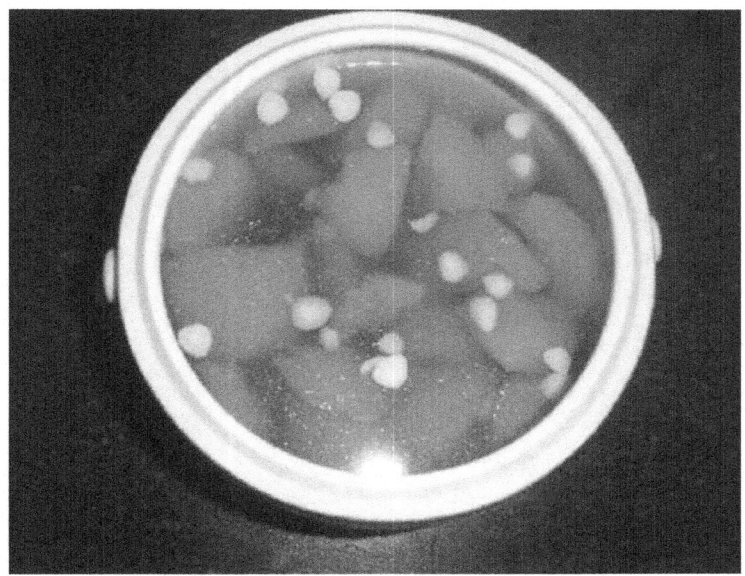

Cooking Time: 43 minutes

Servings: 8

Ingredients:

- ➢ 2 tbsp of olive oil
- ➢ 6 oz of onions, finely chopped
- ➢ 6 oz of dry apricots, quartered (check for foods to avoid)
- ➢ 8 oz of tart apple, peeled and chopped
- ➢ 6 oz of celery, thinly sliced
- ➢ 1 oz of ground almonds
- ➢ 2½ pints boiling water
- ➢ ½ vegetable stock cube (check for foods to avoid)
- ➢ flaked almonds for garnishing

Directions:

1. Heat olive oil; cover and cook celery and onion for about 10 minutes while stirring in between.
2. Mix in ½ stock cube.
3. Add apricots and apple, and cook for 3 more minutes.
4. Add ground almonds, remove it from heat, and then add water.
5. Bring it back to a boil and simmer it covered for around 30 minutes.
6. Place the mixture in blender and blend until smooth.
7. Sprinkle with flaked almonds and serve.

9) Spinach and Carrot Wrap

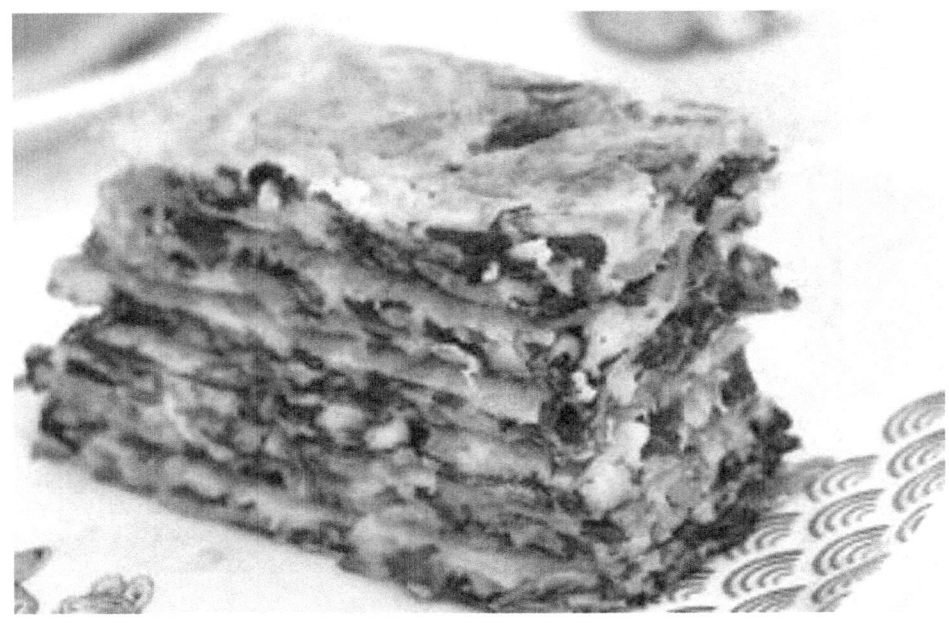

Cooking Time: 12 minutes

Servings: 1

Ingredients:

- 1 tsp of olive oil
- 1 slice of onion
- 1–2 tsps of brown sugar
- 1–2 tsps of molasses
- 1–2 cups of carrots (matchstick carrots are fine)
- 1 handful of spinach
- 1 sprinkle of Italian seasoning or oregano
- Spelt or Ezekiel tortilla (Ezekiel pita bread can also be used.)

Directions:

1. Sauté an onion slice in olive oil.
2. Add carrots; heat them just a little bit.
3. Sprinkle oregano on onion rings and carrots.
4. Add molasses and brown sugar.
5. Heat it for just a little bit.
6. Add 1 handful of spinach.
7. Stir until spinach wilts.
8. Drain and place everything on tortilla and then wrap

10) Kale Crisps

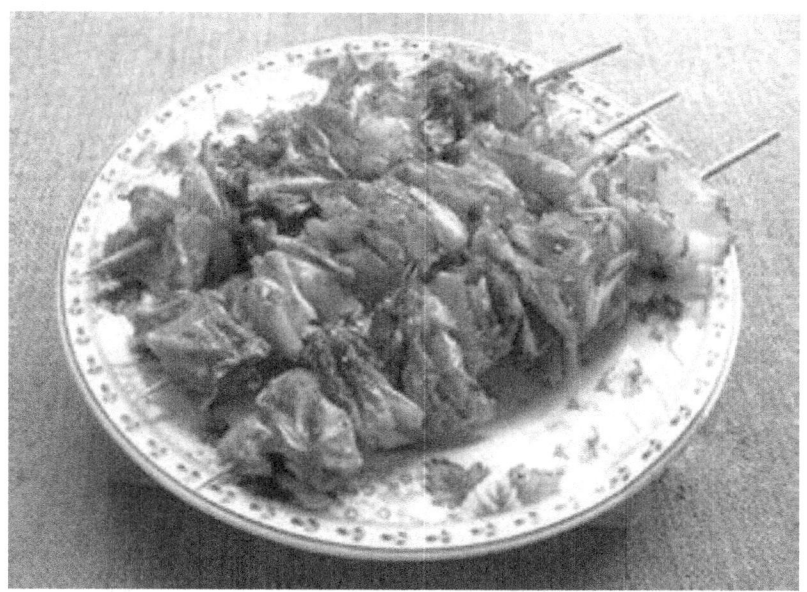

Cooking Time: 20

Servings: 2

Ingredients:

- ➤ 1 bunch of kale
- ➤ 1 pinch of sea salt
- ➤ olive oil cooking spray

Directions:

1. Preheat the oven to 350° F.
2. Rinse and pat dry kale and cut the leaves into bite-size pieces.
3. Line a baking sheet with parchment paper.
4. Spray olive oil generously on kale leaves and toss them with salt.
5. Arrange them in a layer and bake them for about 20 minutes until kale becomes crispy.
6. Enjoy!

Blood Type B Diet Recipes

1) Baked Carrot and Apple Casserole

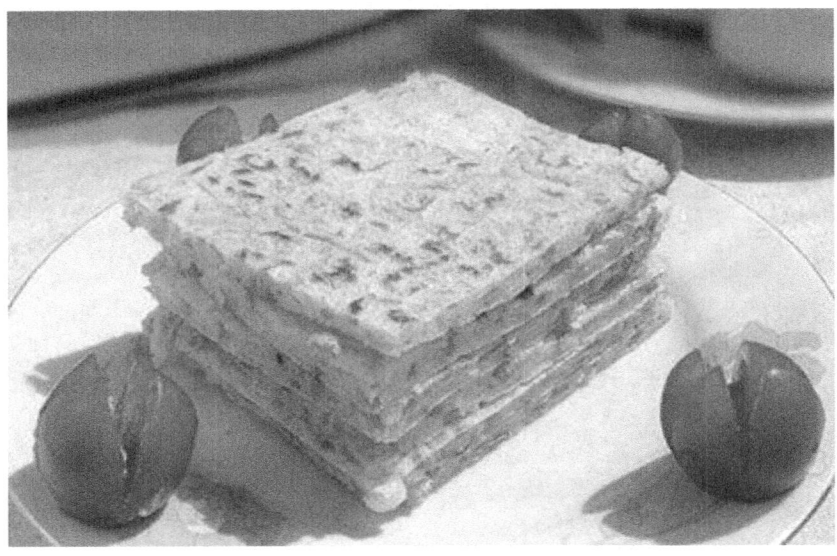

Cooking Time: 45 minutes

Servings: 6

Ingredients:

- 8 apples, peeled, cored, and sliced
- ⅔ quart carrot slices, cooked
- 2⅔ tbsp of white (or whole) spelt flour
- ½ cup of brown sugar (or ¼ cup of agave)
- sea salt, to taste
- 1 cup of lemon juice

Directions:

1. Place half of apple slices in a baking dish and cover them with half of carrot slices.
2. Combine flour, brown sugar, and salt; sprinkle half this mixture over carrot slices.
3. Repeat the layer; pour 1 cup of lemon juice on top.
4. Bake in oven at 350° F for about 45 minutes and serve.

2) Baked Fish Pate

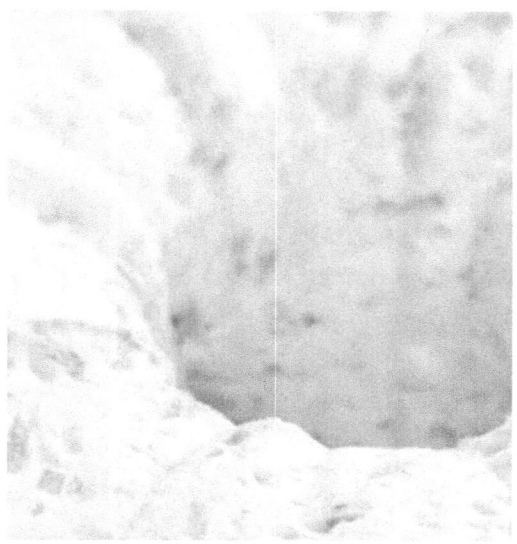

Cooking Time: 45 minutes

Servings: 6

Ingredients:

- ➤ 1 lb of BTD compliance fish fillets, cubed
- ➤ 1 shallot, diced
- ➤ 1 tbsp of lemon zest, grated
- ➤ 1 egg yolk
- ➤ ½–¾ cup of soy milk or regular milk
- ➤ 1 dash of sea salt

Directions:

1. Blend all Ingredients in a blender.
2. Pour it into a greased loaf pan.
3. Place the pan in a bigger pan filled with water.
4. Top it with laurel leaves.
5. Cook in oven at 350° F for about 35–45 minutes or until a toothpick withdraws cleanly.
6. Cool and refrigerate.
7. Slice it and serve with a little bisque poured on each slice.

3) Baked Sweet Potato

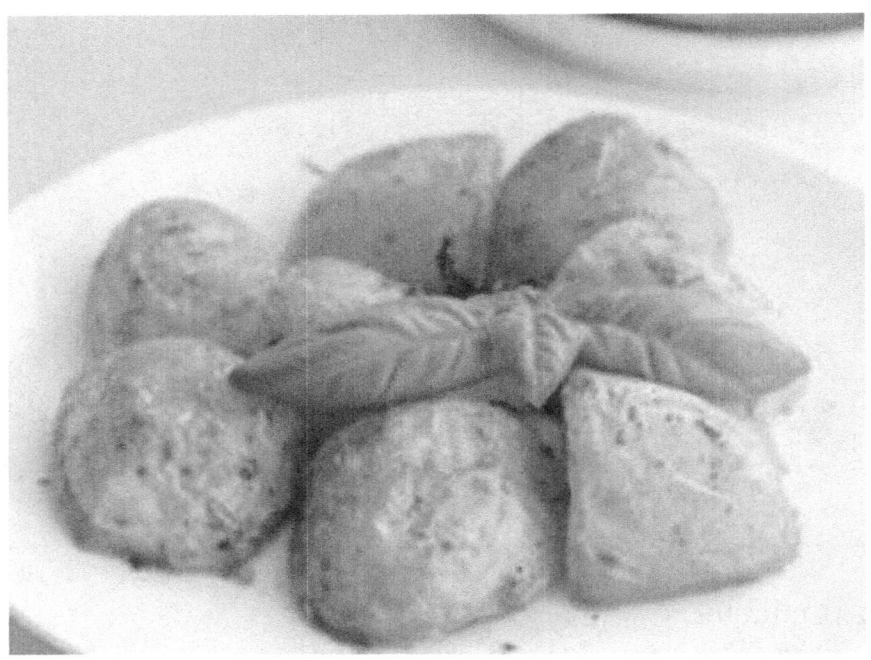

Cooking Time: 1 hour

Servings: 4

Ingredients:

> ➤ 3 large sweet potatoes, peeled and cut into ½-inch slices
> ➤ 2 tbsp of brown sugar
> ➤ ½-inch fresh ginger, cubed into corn-kernel size
> ➤ water

Directions:

1. Arrange the sweet potato slices in layers on bottom of a casserole.
2. Alternate the layers with sprinkles of brown sugar and 1–2 ginger cubes per layer.
3. Pour ½ cup water over whole casserole.
4. Bake it, covered, for about 1 hour in oven heated at 350° F

4) Delicious Beet Greens

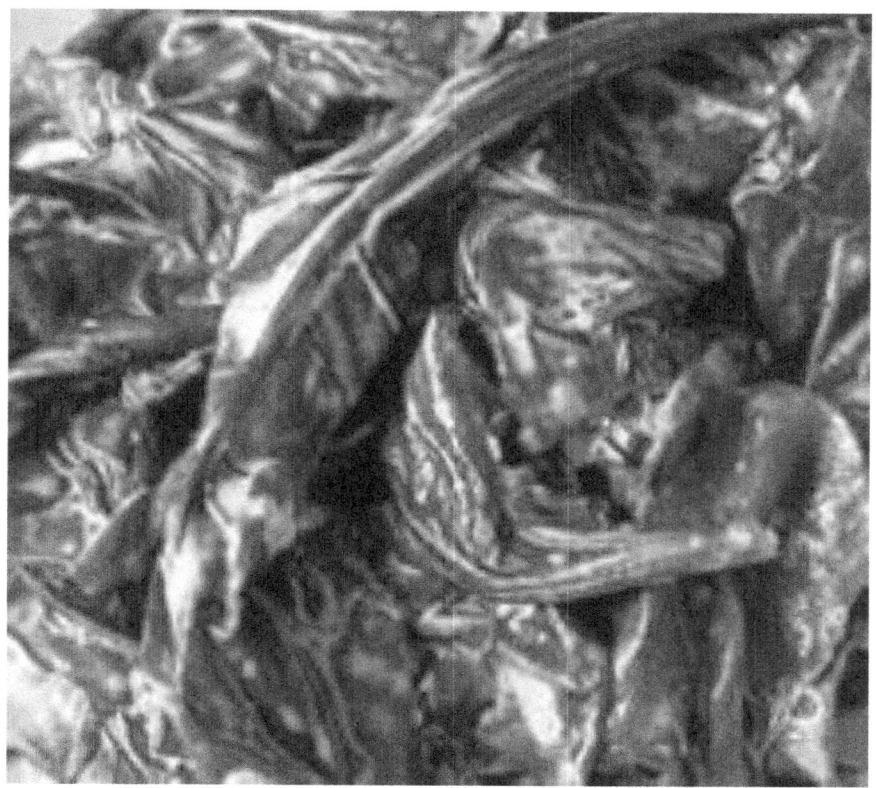

Cooking Time: 15 minutes

Servings: 4

Ingredients:

> ➢ 2 bunches beet greens with whole stems
> ➢ sprinkle powdered cheese or goat feta, to taste
> ➢ granulated garlic, to taste
> ➢ onion, to taste

Directions:

1. Steam beet greens (include stems) in a little bit of water until tender, but do not overcook.
2. Slice across greens and stems into bite-size pieces.
3. Sprinkle powdered cheese or goat feta.
4. Do not add salt (it contains enough of its own).
5. Add a little onion or granulated garlic for extra punch for the immune system.

5) Better Flax Biscuits

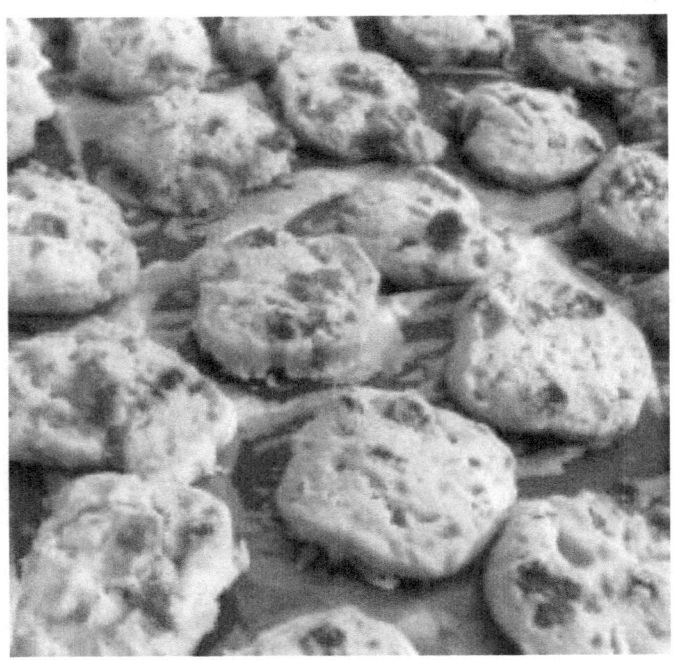

Cooking Time: 30 minutes

Servings: 5

Ingredients:

- ➢ 1 cup of rice flour
- ➢ 1 cup of golden flax meal
- ➢ 2 tbsp of ghee
- ➢ 1 tsp of baking powder
- ➢ 2 tbsp of vegetable glycerine
- ➢ ¾ cup of hot water

Directions:

1. Preheat the oven at 350° F.
2. Gently combine all Ingredients together.
3. Spoon out the mixture onto a greased baking sheet; bake for about 20–25 minutes.
4. To prepare cobbler topping, place 1 can crushed pineapple in a bowl (or 3–4 cups other fruit, along with a little bit of juice or water).
5. Squeeze a little bit of honey, agave, or vegetable glycerine over top.
6. Spoon this topping on biscuits and bake until biscuits are done.

6) Blueberry Vanilla–Flavoured Cookies

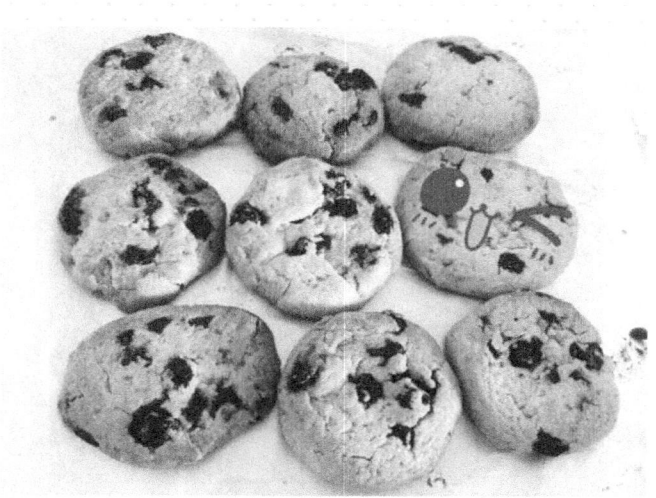

Cooking Time: 14 minutes

Yields: 10 cookies

Ingredients:

- ➤ 1 heaping tbsp of ghee
- ➤ 1 tbsp of rice milk or any BTD-compliant milk
- ➤ ⅔ cup of brown sugar (or any BTD-compliant sugar substitute]
- ➤ 1 tsp of real vanilla
- ➤ ½ tsp of baking powder
- ➤ ¼ tsp of sea salt, fine crystals
- ➤ ¼ cup of applesauce (or 1 egg)
- ➤ 1 cup of millet flour or ½ cup of oat flour plus ½ cup of brown rice flour
- ➤ ¼ cup of fresh blueberries (frozen also work)

Directions:

1. Cream ghee with sugar.
2. Add vanilla and milk and beat.
3. Beat in remaining Ingredients except blueberries.
4. Fold in the blueberries gently.
5. Drop the mixture using a teaspoon onto a non-stick baking sheet.
6. Bake them at 350° F for about 10–14 minutes.
7. Let the cookies completely cool before removing.

7) Flax Oats Muffins

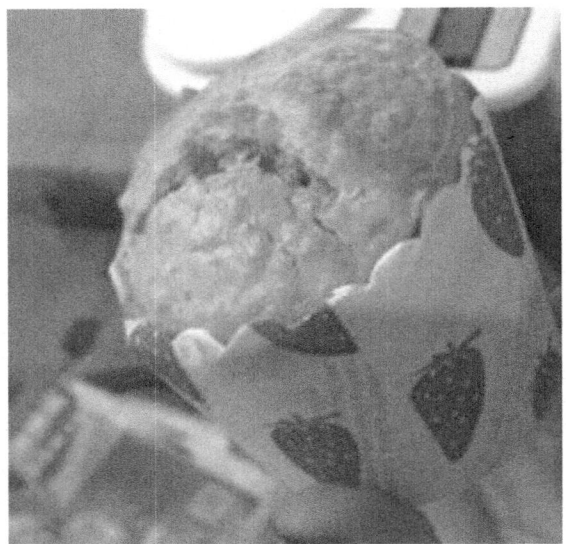

Cooking Time: 18 minutes

Servings: 6

Ingredients:

- 3 cups of ground flax seed (golden)
- ¾ cup of milk (½ cup of rice milk and ¼ cup of soy milk)
- 1¼ cup of flour (¾ cup each of oats and spelt)
- ½ cup of sweetener (molasses)
- 2 tbsp of oil (1 tbsp each of sesame and olive)
- 1 tbsp of baking powder
- 2 large eggs
- 1 dash cinnamon (optional)
- 1 dash sea salt (optional)

- 1 tsp almond or vanilla extract (optional)

Directions:

1. Preheat the oven to 350° F.
2. Mix all the dry Ingredients in a bowl and all wet Ingredients in another.
3. Beat them up.
4. Mix dry Ingredients and wet Ingredients together.
5. Spoon this mixture onto greased muffin pan
6. Bake them for about 18 minutes.

8) Millet Veggie Bread

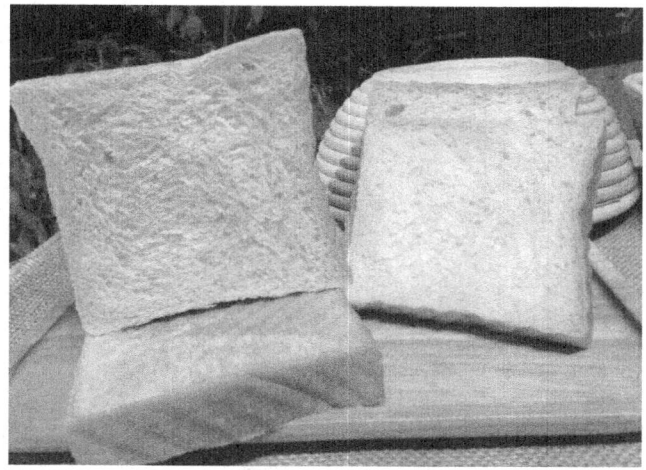

Cooking Time: 1 hour

Servings: 4

Ingredients:

> ➢ 1 cup of whole millet
> ➢ 1 cup of yogurt
> ➢ 3 eggs
> ➢ 1 cup of water
> ➢ 1 tsp of sea salt (real or Celtic)
> ➢ 1 tbsp of ghee

Optional Ingredients:

> ➢ 1 cup of zucchini
> ➢ 1 cup of red onion
> ➢ 1 cup of other vegetables (broccoli, spinach, Swiss chard, etc.)
> ➢ 1 cup of BTD-compliant cheese

Directions:

1. Coat the baking dish using ghee
2. Mix remaining Ingredients; pour in a baking dish.
3. Bake it in oven on 375° F for about 1 hour.

9) Quinoa Muffins

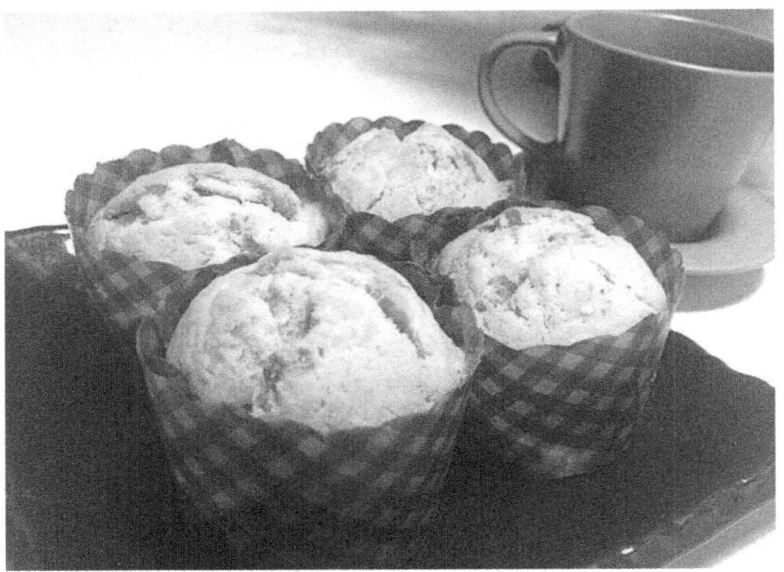

Cooking Time: 30 minutes

Servings: 6 (3 muffins per serving)

Ingredients:

- ➢ 1 cup of rice flour (or spelt flour)
- ➢ 1½ cup of quinoa flour (or 1 cup of quinoa flour + ½ cup of millet flour)
- ➢ 1 tsp of baking powder
- ➢ 1 tsp of baking soda
- ➢ 2 tsp of sea salt
- ➢ 2 eggs, beaten
- ➢ ¼ cup of ghee (or butter), softened
- ➢ 2 cups of desired milk according to blood type rice, nut, or soy milk plus a little bit of lemon juice or plain yogurt

Directions:

1. Preheat the oven to 425° F.
2. Sift together dry Ingredients.
3. Cut ghee until the mixture resembles bread crumbs.
4. Combine milk and eggs, and then stir it into flour mixture.
5. Bake in oven in greased muffin pan for about 25–30 minutes.

10) Soy Oatmeal Cookies (High Protein)

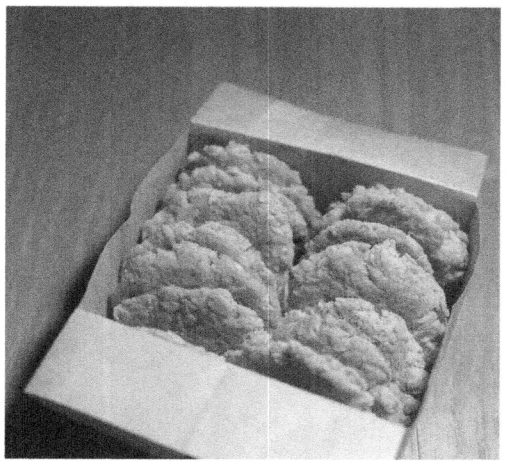

Cooking Time: 10–12 minutes

Servings: 6

Ingredients:

- 1½ cups of all-purpose or any BTD-compliant flour
- ¾ cup of soybean flour
- 2 cups of oatmeal
- 1 tsp of baking powder
- 1 tsp of salt
- 1 cup of compliant oil
- 1 cup of granulated sugar
- ¾ cup of brown sugar
- 2 eggs
- 1 tsp of vanilla
- ½ cup of water
- 1 tsp of nutmeg
- 1 cup of raisins or dry cherries (optional)

Directions:

1. Combine baking powder, the flours, oatmeal, salt, and spices in a bowl.
2. In another mixing bowl, mix sugar and oil.
3. Add vanilla and eggs to creamed mixture; beat for about 2 minutes.
4. Add the flour mixture gradually, stir in raisins or cherries, and mix well.
5. Drop the mixture using rounded spoons onto the greased baking sheet. Press them down slightly with a fork.
6. Bake in oven at 350° F for about 10 minutes to get chewy cookies and for about 12 minutes to get crunchy cookies.

Blood Type AB Diet Recipes

1) Potato Tuna Salad

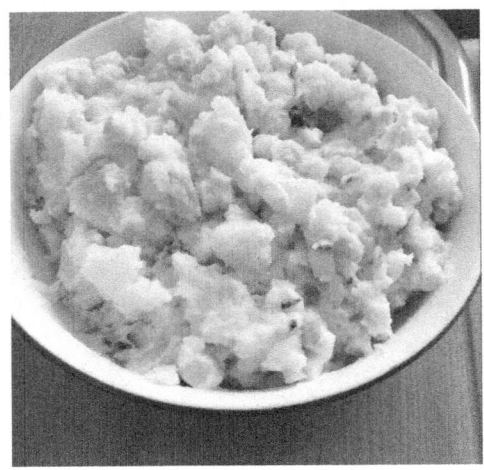

Cooking Time: 45 minutes - 50 minutes

Yield: 1-2 Serving(s)

Ingredients:

> - 1 jar of canned tuna
> - 2 small Potatoes
> - ½ cucumber
> - ½ carrot
> - 1 tbsp. Milk
> - ¼ cup corn
> - Italian vinaigrette salad dressing to taste
> - Salt to taste
> - Black pepper to taste

Directions:

1) Peel, wash and cut the potato into small cubes, cook them in boiled water for 15mins-20 mins (Insert a fork into the potatoes, if potatoes are fully cooked, it will be easy for the forks to piece the potatoes.)
2) Wash and Dice the cucumber and carrots, drain the tuna
3) Mash the potato with a spoon
4) Mix milk, salt and black pepper into mashed potato. Stir well
5) Stir-fry the corns in a skillet until fully cooked. Drain the corns on paper towel
6) Combine corns, carrot cubes, cucumber cubes, and tuna into the mashed potato.
7) Add Italian vinaigrette salad dressing and honey, stir well.

2) Broccoli Salad

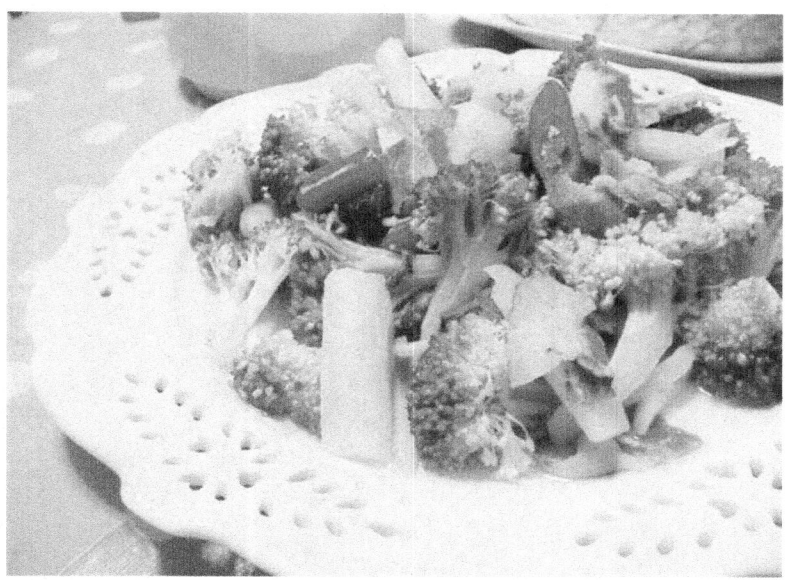

Prep Time: 10 minutes + 8 hours refrigerating time

Servings: 8

Ingredients:

- 2 large heads broccoli, cut into small pieces
- ½–1 cup of raisins
- ¼–½ fake bacon bits (soy based or anything that fits your profile)

Dressing:

- ⅓–½ cup of mayonnaise
- 2 tbsp of lemon juice
- 2 tbsp of sugar
- ½ cup of sunflower seeds or sliced almond

Directions:

1. Prepare dressing by combining all dressing Ingredients and allowing it to sit while broccoli is prepared.
2. Pour the dressing over broccoli pieces, raisins, and fake bacon bits
3. Stir well to evenly distribute dressing and allow it to sit overnight in refrigerator. Dressing melds well as it sits.
4. Sprinkle nuts and toss well just prior to serving.

3) Quick Zucchini Salad

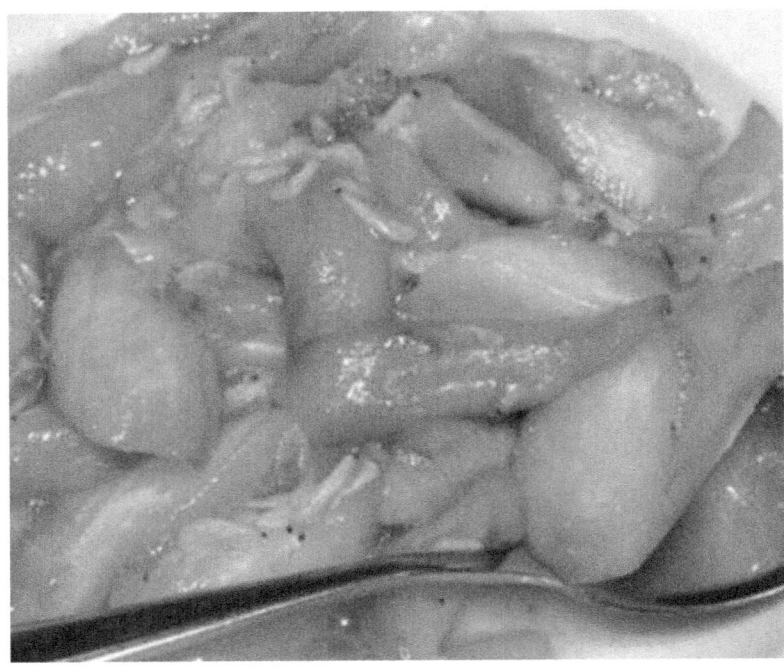

Prep Time: 10 minutes + Marinating Time

Servings: 1

Ingredients:

- ➢ 1 medium zucchini
- ➢ 2 oz of feta cheese
- ➢ 1 tbsp of olive oil (or more)
- ➢ 1 tbsp of lime or lemon juice (Type B people can use balsamic vinegar)

Directions:

1. Cut the zucchini lengthwise into quarters and chop coarsely.
2. Crumble 2 oz of feta cheese over top.
3. Whip oil and lime or lemon juice together.
4. Pour it over feta and zucchini. Toss gently.
5. Serve immediately or allow it to marinate for a couple of hours.

4) Pumpkin Salad

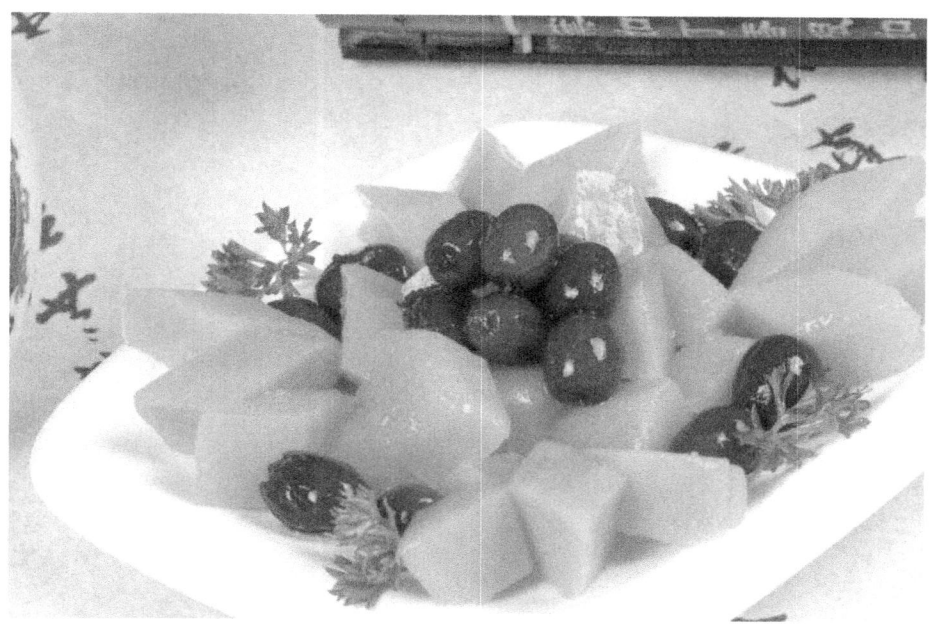

Prep Time: 10 minutes

Cook Time: 10 minutes

Servings: 1

Ingredients:

- ➢ 100 g of pumpkin
- ➢ 2 tsp of virgin olive oil
- ➢ 1 tsp of honey
- ➢ 2 oz of feta cheese, crumbled
- ➢ A handful of pine nuts

Directions:

1. Cut the pumpkin into bite-size pieces
2. Drizzle with honey and olive oil.
3. Roast in oven until cooked, for about 10 minutes.
4. Remove it from oven; place it into serving bowl; toss with toasted feta cheese and pine nuts.
5. Serve it is as a salad or along with pasta/orzo as a main dish.

5) Spelt and Flax Bread

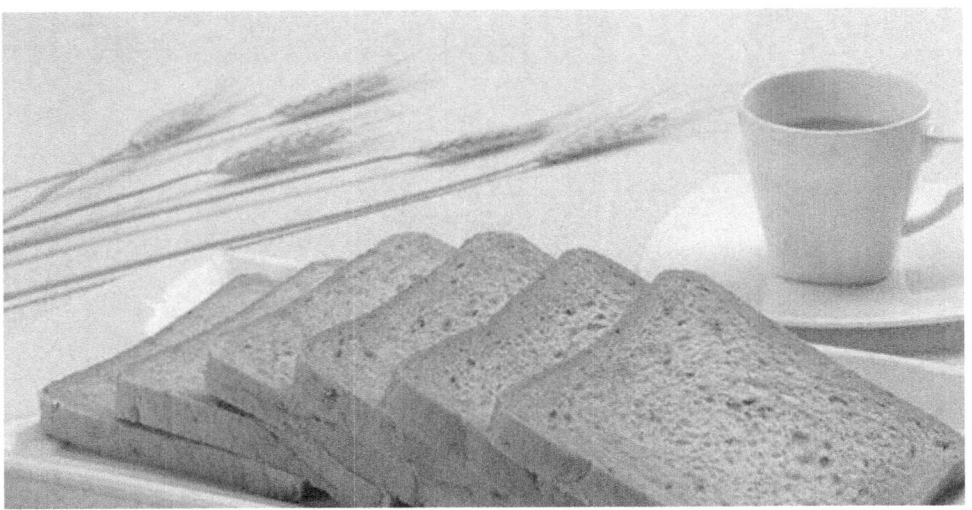

Cooking Time: 55 minutes

Yields: 3 loafs

Ingredients:

- 3 cups of warm water
- 1 tbsp of instant yeast
- ⅓ cup of olive oil
- 1 tbsp of sea salt
- 1 egg
- ⅓–⅔ cup of honey (depending on desired sweetness)
- 7 cups of flour (1 cup of brown rice flour, ⅓ cup of flax meal, 1 cup of whole spelt, and the rest white spelt)

Directions:

1. Combine water, oil, egg, and honey.
2. Add salt, flour, and yeast and knead for 3–5 minutes.
3. Knead the surface with ⅓ cup of olive oil to keep the dough moist.
4. Cover it and let it rise until double.
5. Place the dough into 3 greased loaf pans.
6. Bake at 200° F for about 25 minutes and then turn up the heat to 350° F for about 30 minutes or until done.

6) Spinach and Yogurt Dip

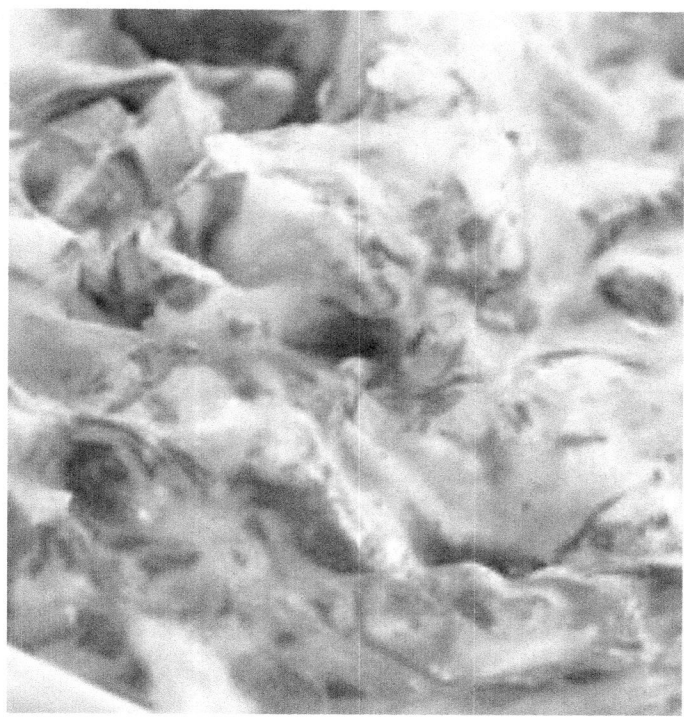

Prep Time: 10 minutes

Servings: 6

Ingredients:

- ➤ 1 (32 oz) can of plain yogurt
- ➤ 1 box of chopped spinach, frozen
- ➤ 1 dash of sugar (optional)
- ➤ 1 tsp of mayonnaise (optional)
- ➤ 1 dash of sea salt
- ➤ 1 tsp more of cayenne pepper
- ➤ 1 tsp of cumin
- ➤ 1 tsp of curry powder

Directions:

1. In a colander, place a paper towel. Add yogurt and let it drain for 3–4 hours in refrigerator.
2. Return it to a bowl and add spinach and remaining Ingredients. Add in spices and adjust them, to taste.

7) Tofu Egg Salad

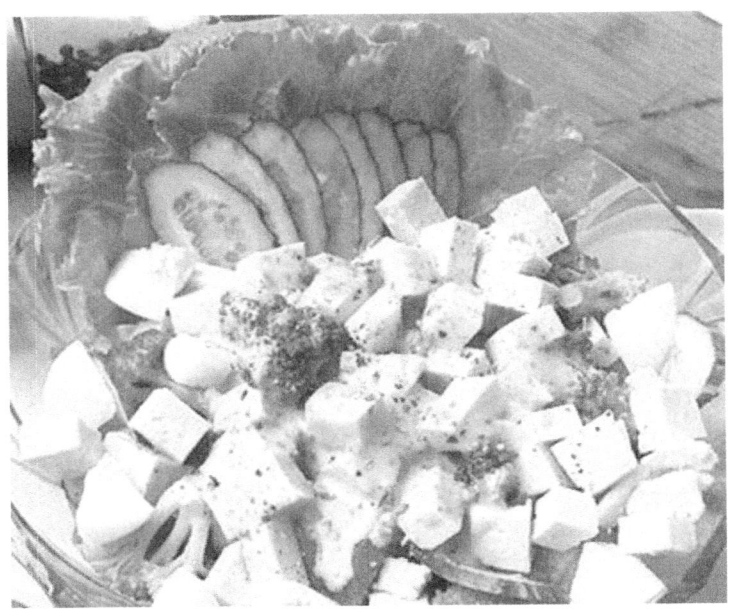

Prep Time: 10 minutes

Servings: 2

Ingredients:-

- ½ lb of tofu
- 1 scallion chopped
- 2 tbsp of mayonnaise
- ½ cucumber, diced
- 1 tbsp of tahini
- 1 dash of salt
- 1 dash of pepper
- 1 tbsp of prepared mustard
- 1 dash of garlic powder

Directions:

1. In a bowl, mash tofu using a fork.
2. Add mayo, tahini, seasonings, mustard, and chopped vegetables.
3. Mix well using spoon.
4. Serve it cold.

8) Walnut Apple Muffins

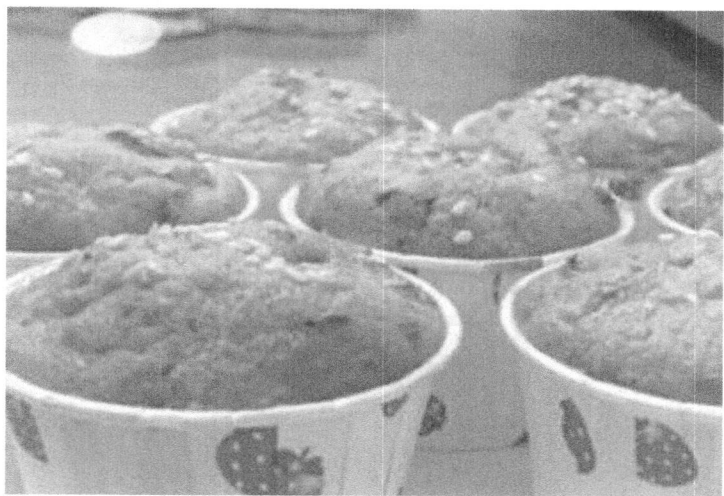

Cooking Time: 12 minutes

Servings: 12

Ingredients:

- 1½ cups of rye flour (or ¾ cup of each of rye flour and spelt flour)
- 2 tbsp of arrowroot powder
- 2 tsp of baking powder
- 1 tsp of cinnamon
- ¼ tsp of sea salt
- ½–1 cup of walnuts, chopped
- 3 tbsp of soy milk
- 1 tbsp of extra-light olive oil
- 1 tbsp of honey (or agave syrup)
- ¾ cup of stewed apple-raisin mix

Directions:

1. Preheat the oven to 425°F.
2. Grease a muffin tin with olive oil.
3. Sift the flour; add baking powder, arrowroot, cinnamon, nuts, and salt in a mixing bowl.
4. Make a dig; add soy milk, apple mix, and sweetener.
5. Mix gently, adding additional liquid 2 tbsp at a time until flour gets moistened.
6. Evenly divide dough into 12 muffins cups and bake them for around 12 minutes.
7. Immediately after taking out from oven, loosen the muffins; turn them sideways in the cups for cooling.

9) Gluten-Free Flax and Millet Crackers

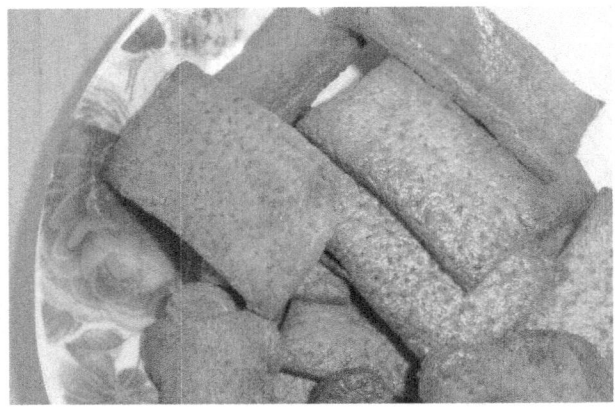

Cooking Time: 25 minutes

Servings: 6

Ingredients:

- ½ cup of flax meal (or another ½ cup millet/rice flour)
- 1½ cup of millet flour or rice flour
- 1 tsp of baking soda
- ½ tsp of onion powder
- ½ tsp of garlic powder
- 2 tsp of Italian herbs (oregano, basil, etc.)
- 1 tsp of turmeric
- 1 tsp of sea salt
- 1 cup of desired cheese, grated
- 4–5 tbsp of water
- 3 tbsp of ghee, oil or butter

Directions:

1. Preheat the oven to 350° F.
2. Line the baking sheet with parchment paper.
3. Mix Ingredients in the bowl with hands.
4. Place the dough on the parchment paper; press the dough flat with oiled. Try to get ¼-inch thickness.
5. Using a metal spatula, cut dough into squares of desired size. Press them down and wiggle them slightly; press them down again.
6. Bake them for about 15–25 minutes.
7. Remove them, cool, and serve.

10) Lemony Shortbread Bars

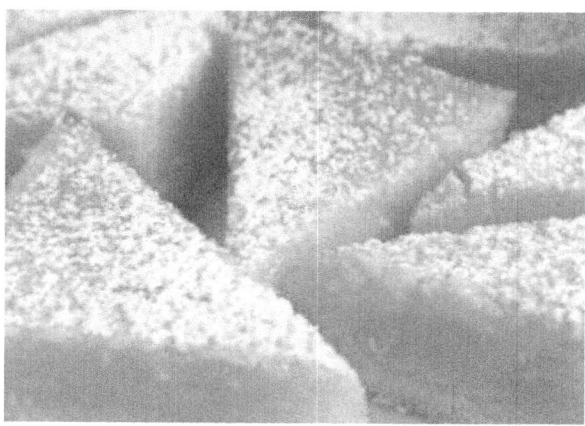

Cooking Time: 30 minutes

Yields: 1 loaf

Ingredients:

For Shortbread:

- 2 tbsp of agave
- 1 ⅓ cup of spelt flour (or rice flour)
- ½ cup of butter, softened

For Lemon topping:

- ⅔ cup of agave
- 2 tbsp of arrowroot starch
- 2 egg yolks
- ¼ cup of water
- 3 tbsp of lemon juice
- 1 tbsp of butter

Directions:

1. Preheat the oven to 325° F.
2. Cream butter and agave together; add spelt flour; pour it into a baking pan.
3. Evenly spread the mixture using a spoon; bake for about 25–30 minutes.
4. While shortbread bakes, mix agave, water, and starch in a pan over medium-low heat until bubbly.
5. Add lemon juice and egg yolks (beaten); cook for about 2–3 more minutes.
6. Remove it from heat; add butter while stirring until mixed.
7. Pour this lemon topping on baked shortbread, cover it, and cool it in refrigerator for about 20–30 min.

11) Lemon and Poppy seed Muffins

Cooking Time: 20 minutes

Yields: 12 muffins

Ingredients:

- ➢ 1 cup of hot water
- ➢ 1 cup of golden flax meal (or regular flax meal)
- ➢ 1 tsp (or more) lemon peel, grated
- ➢ 1 tbsp of fresh lemon juice
- ➢ 1 tbsp of ghee, oil or butter
- ➢ 1 cup of millet or rice flour
- ➢ 1 tsp of baking soda
- ➢ 8 tbsp of honey or agave
- ➢ ½ tsp of salt
- ➢ 1 tbsp of poppy seeds

Directions:

1. Preheat the oven to 325° F.
2. Line a muffin tin using paper cups.
3. Heat water.
4. Stir in flax meal until smooth and thick.
5. Stir in remaining liquid Ingredients.
6. Mix dry Ingredients.
7. Stir everything together and divide it among 12 muffin cups.
8. Bake them for about 20 minutes.
9. Allow the muffins to completely cool and serve.

Blood Type O Diet Recipes

1) Sweet and Sour Fish

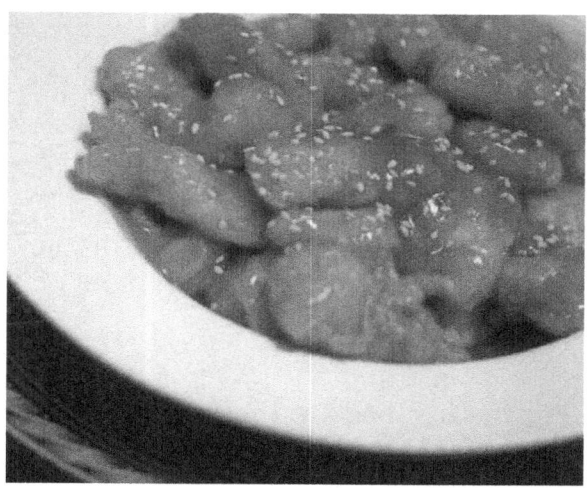

Cooking Time: 35 minutes

Yield: 2 **Servings**

Ingredients:

- 2 cup chopped fish fillet
- 2 tbsp. chopped Onion
- ½ tbsp. chopped Ginger (optional)
- 1 tablespoon chicken stock
- 1/2 tsp salt
- 1/4 teaspoon pepper
- Sweet and sour sauce:
- 3 tablespoons white vinegar
- 3 tablespoons white sugar
- 2 tablespoons tomato paste
- 2 tsp salt
- 3 tablespoons water
- 1 tsp. Starch
- 2-3 cups frying oil
- 1 tbsp. olive oil
- Sesame seeds for garnishing

Step 1

Wash the fish fillets and cut into cubes

Step 2

Marinate fish cubes with 1 tsp. salt, pepper for 20 minutes.

Step 3

Dice onion, ginger, set aside. Mix vinegar, sugar, tomato paste, 1 tsp. salt, water and starch together. Set aside.

Step 4

Dip fish into starch

Step 5

Heat a pan or a pot with 2-4 cups of frying oil (cover most of the fish fillets), deep fry the fish cubes until they turn white. Spoon the fish out and place them on a paper towel.

Step 6

Turn up the fire on high; Put the fish back to the pot/pan and deep fry the fish again until golden brown.

Step 7

Take another pan, add 3 tbsp. olive oil and turn fire on medium low, throw onions and ginger in the pan, fry them until they are slightly browned. Spoon the fish fillet cubes out and drain the oil on paper towel.

Step 8

Pour the sweet and sour sauce into the pan, turn up the fire on high and stir until the sauce is thicken.

Step 9

Pour the fish into the pan and stir fry them for 30 seconds to 1 minutes, make sure all the fish are covered with the sweet and sour sauce.

Garnish with sesame seeds.

Tips

Add ketchup into sweet and sour sauce can make the color of the dish look prettier and the taste richer. If you don't like ketchup, you can just omit it like I do.

Don't heat the sweet and sour sauce for too long. Vinegar evaporates faster than sugar. If you heat up the sauce for too long, the dish might end up with only sweet flavour.

2) Artichoke and Spinach Dip

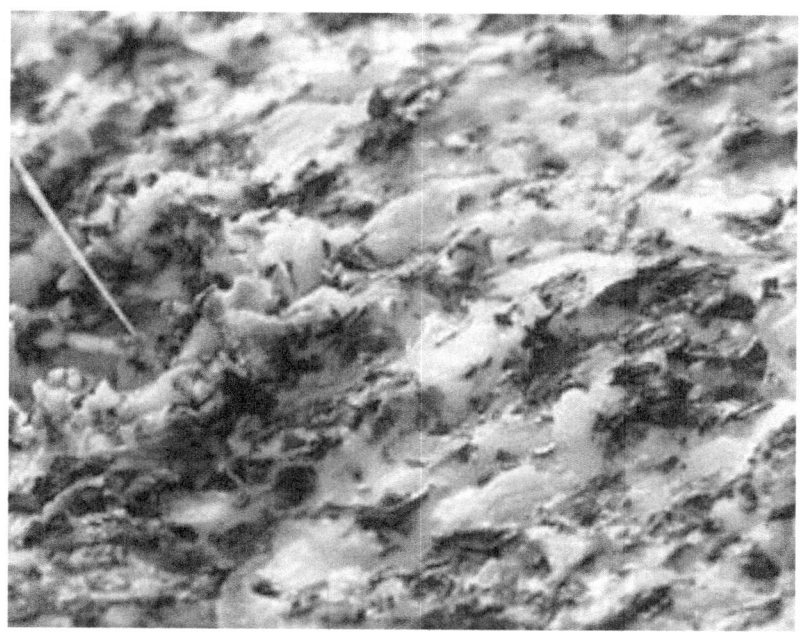

Prep Time: 5 minutes

Servings: 6

Ingredients:

- ➢ 1 can artichoke hearts
- ➢ Fresh spinach
- ➢ 1 tsp of garlic, minced
- ➢ 1 dash of sea salt
- ➢ Dairy-free mayonnaise (or other BTD-compliant mayonnaise)

Directions:

Drain the artichoke hearts; add all the Ingredients; puree them in the blender.

3) Simple Japanese Salmon

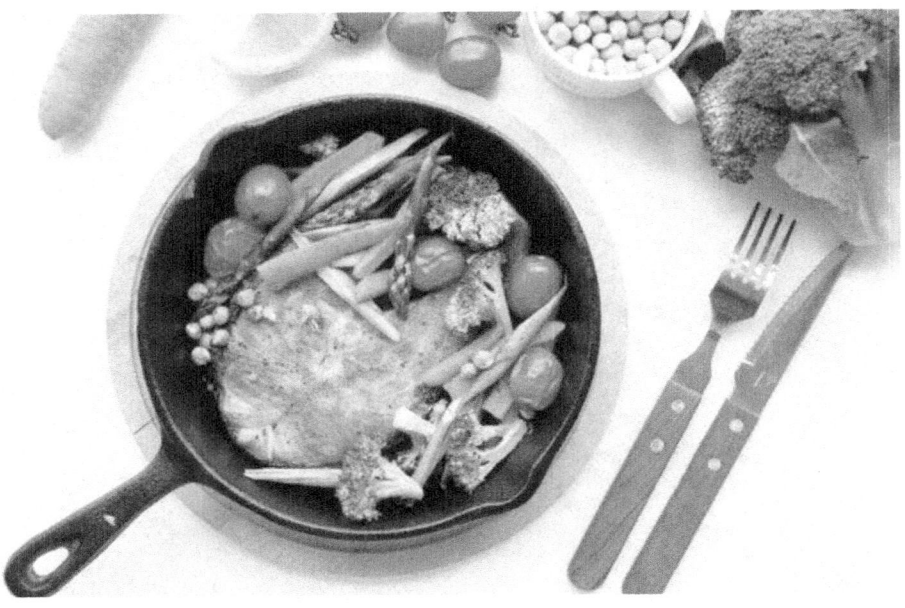

Cooking Time: 8 minutes (Marinate 24-48 hours)

Yield: 1-2 serving (s)

Ingredients:

> ➢ Large size Salmon fillet (avoid smoked salmon) 1 piece
> ➢ Salt.

Direction:

1. Cover both side of salmon with salt and marinate for 24 - 48 hours (make sure the ice and water are removed before marinate)
2. Place salmon in a skillet (non-stick, don't put oil in the skillet) on medium fire, cook until both sides of the salmon become golden brown,(about 8 minutes- we want to cook salmon in this dish for longer time)
3. Serve with sautéed vegetables

4) Smoky Beef-Brisket

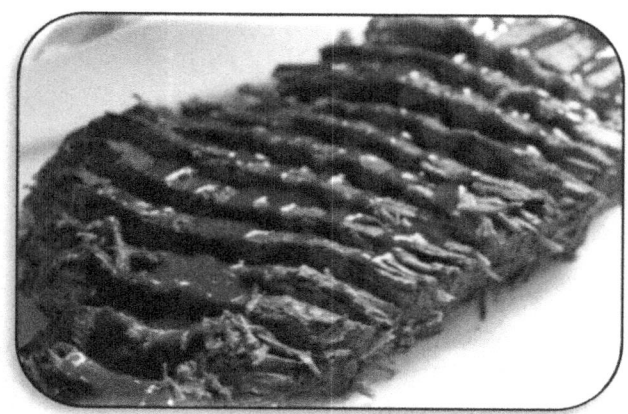

Cook Time: 1h25mins

Servings: 6

Ingredients:-

> - 3 lb of beef brisket, fat-trimmed, flat cut
> - 1 tsp of seasoned meat tenderizer
> - ¼ tsp of Lowry's seasoned salt
> - ¼ tsp of garlic salt
> - ¼ tsp of celery salt(Can be substituted with ¼ tsp regular salt)
> - 1 tbsp of Worcester sauce
> - 2 tbsp of liquid smoke
> - ½ cup of water
> - 1 cup of BBQ sauce, plus extra to serve

Directions:-

1. Mix beef, seasoned salt, garlic salt and celery salt (or ¼ tsp regular salt) in a bowl. Massage the spices into the brisket. Put the brisket in a Ziploc bag. Add Worcester sauce and liquid smoke. Seal the bag and put it in refrigerator for overnight to marinate.
2. Put BBQ sauce and water in the pressure cooker. Add brisket along with any juices from bag in the cooker. Cook on high pressure for60 minutes.(If using stove top pressure cooker, cook for 10-20 minutes on high heat until reaches the pressure, then turn down the fire to medium low) When time is up, remove from heat and let pressure release naturally for about 15 minutes and carefully remove the lid. Carefully remove meat from pressure cooker into a plate and slice the meat.
3. Serve and enjoy

5) BBQ Meatballs

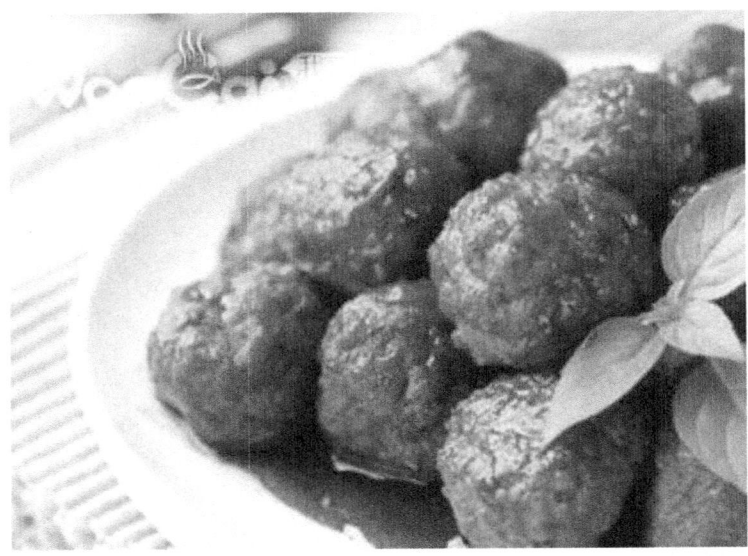

This is an easy-to-make and delicious party snacks. It's made with only 3 Ingredients.

Cook Time: 10-15 minutes

Servings: 7 (Yields 42 meatballs)

Ingredients:-

> ➤ 1 bag (48 oz) of beef meatballs (frozen and fully cooked)
> ➤ 18 oz of BBQ Sauce
> ➤ 18 oz of grape jelly

Directions:-

1. Add a cup of water to the cooking pot. Place steamer basket in cooking pot; add meatballs. Cook them for 5 minutes at high pressure. When time is up, release pressure using quick release method. Take out the steamer basket from cooking pot and remove meatballs.
2. Discard the cooking water; add grape jelly and BBQ sauce to the cooking pot. Simmer the sauce in the pressure cooker with open lid on medium high fire, stirring regularly. Add meatballs when jelly and barbecue sauce combines together and becomes smooth. Stir well.
3. Serve and Enjoy.

6) Almond Flax muffins

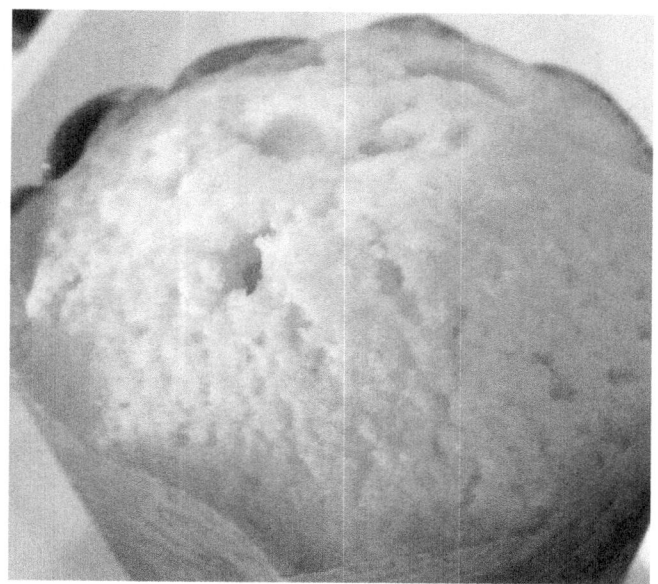

Cooking Time: 20 minutes

Servings: 8 rolls

Ingredients:

- 1½ cups of almond flour
- 1 cup of ground flax
- 1½ tsp of baking powder
- ½ tsp of baking soda
- 3 eggs
- ¼–½ tsp of sea salt (to taste)
- ¼–½ cup of water

Directions:

1. Preheat the oven to 350° F.
2. Grease the muffin pan with non-stick spray or oil.
3. Combine all the dry Ingredients in one bowl.
4. In a separate bowl, mix the wet Ingredients.
5. Add the wet Ingredients with the dry Ingredients and combine well.
6. Wait for a couple of minutes as flax causes the batter to become thick.
7. Spoon it into the prepared muffin pan, each muffin tin around ¾ full.
8. Bake them at 350° F for about 20 minutes or until toothpick inserted withdraws cleanly.
9. Cool the muffins on a rack.

7) Amaranth and Quinoa Gingerbread Muffins

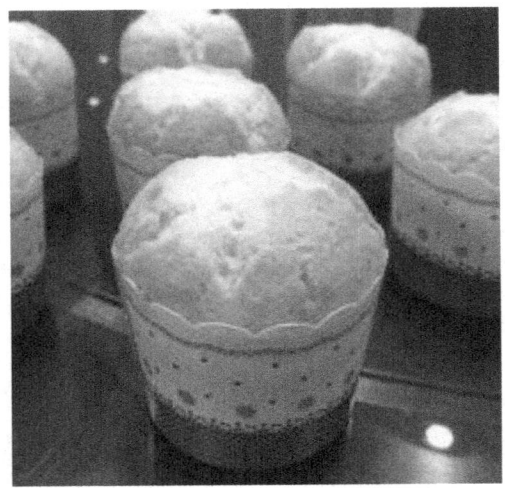

Cooking Time: 30 minutes

Yields: 18 muffins

Ingredients:

- ½ cup of amaranth flour
- 1¼ cups of quinoa flour
- ½ cup of rice flour
- ¼ cup of flaxseed meal
- ½ cup of millet flour (or BTD-compliant substitute)
- 1 tsp of baking soda
- 1 tsp of baking powder
- 2 tsp of sea salt
- 2 tsp of ginger
- ½ tsp of cinnamon (or BTD-compliant substitute)
- ½ tsp of cardamom
- ½ tsp of cloves
- ¼ cup of ghee or BTD-compliant oil
- ¼ cup of blackstrap molasses
- 2 cups of liquid (milk, nut milk, yogurt, or water)
- 2 eggs

Directions:

1. Preheat the oven to 425° F.
2. Sift together the dry Ingredients.
3. Cut in ghee (if using) until mixture resembles bread crumbs.
4. Combine eggs, molasses, and milk, and then stir liquids into flour mixture.
5. Bake it in greased muffin pan for about 25–30 minutes.

8) Blueberry and Buckwheat Bread

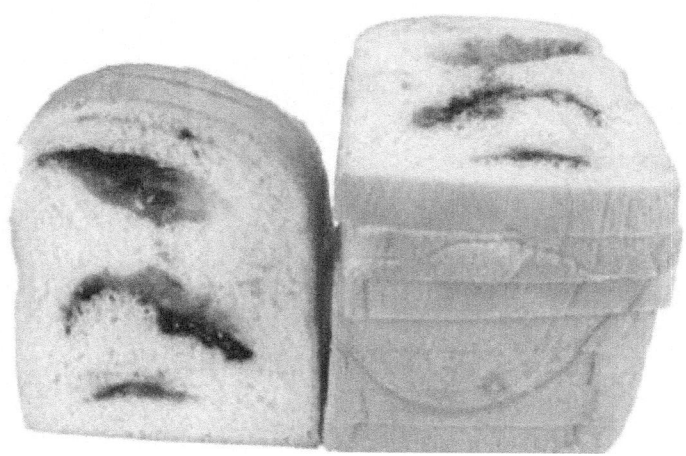

Cooking Time: 1½ hour

Yields: 1 loaf (16 slices)

Ingredients:

- ¾ cup of barley flour (100 percent organic)
- ¾ cup of buckwheat flour
- 1 cup of pure cane sugar (or Sucanat sugar)
- 1 cup of blueberries (fresh or frozen)
- 2 tsp of baking powder
- ¼ cup of canola oil (organic)
- ½ cup of walnuts, chopped
- 1 cup of unsweetened applesauce (organic)
- ½ lemon juice and boiling water (to make 1 cup of liquid)
- 3 egg whites

Directions:

1. Preheat the oven to 325° F.
2. Mix together the dry Ingredients and keep aside.
3. Grate the lemon zest and reserve; squeeze out ½ cup of lemon juice.
4. Add sufficient boiling water to lemon juice to make one cup of liquid.
5. Combine lemon juice and zest with remaining Ingredients.
6. Mix well and pour it in a lightly greased (soybean) loaf pan.
7. Bake it for about 1½ hours (or until knife inserted at centre withdraws cleanly).

9) Carrot Muffins

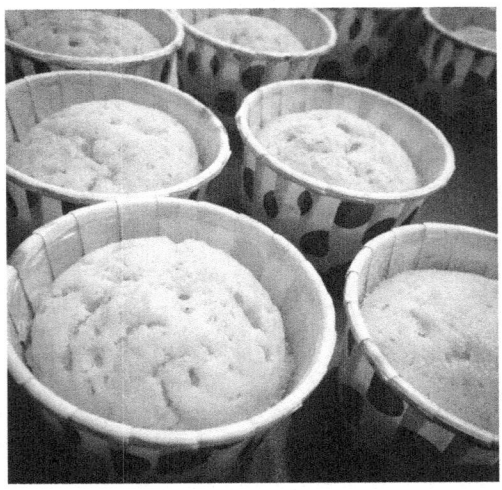

Cooking Time: 20 minutes

Yields: 12 muffins

Ingredients:

- 125 g of Olivine
- ¼ cup of brown sugar
- ¾ cup of sugar
- 2 eggs
- 1½ cups of gluten-free flour mix (or BTD-compliant substitute)
- ½ tsp of sea salt
- 2 tsp of baking powder
- 2 tsp of mixed spice
- ½ cup of sultanas (optional), grated
- ½ cup of walnuts, chopped
- 250 g of carrot (approximately 1 cup)
- 1 tsp of cinnamon
- ½ tsp of ground nutmeg
- ¼ tsp of ground clove
- ½ tsp of ginger
- 50 g of finely chopped dry pineapple (optional)

Directions:

1. Preheat the oven to 350° F.
2. Line the muffin tin using paper.
3. Beat butter, eggs, and sugars together.
4. Mix in remaining Ingredients.
5. Divide the mixture into muffin liners.
6. Bake them for about 18–20 minutes.
7. Cool them in tin until cold.

10) Gingerbread

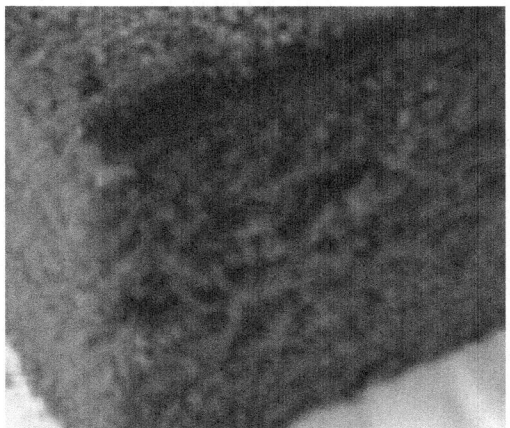

Cooking Time: 12 minutes

Yields: 10 (6-8 inch) gingerbreads

Ingredients:

- 100 g or ½ cup of butter (or ghee)
- 85 g or ⅓ cup of agave, or 110 g or ½ cup of sugar
- 405 g or 3¼ cups of amaranth flour, sifted
- 1 tsp of sea salt
- 1 tsp of baking soda
- ½ tsp of ground allspice/cloves/cinnamon
- 1 tsp of ground ginger
- 180 mL or ¾ cup of molasses
- 60 mL or ¼ cup of water

Directions:

1. Cream the butter with agave in a bowl.
2. In another bowl, sift the flour with baking soda, sea salt, and spices.
3. Blend the flour mixture into the creamed mixture alternately with water and molasses and make sure each is incorporated completely before adding next.
4. Chill for a minimum of 1 hour.
5. Preheat the oven to 350° F.
6. Roll the dough into ¼-inch thickness. Cut it with gingerbread men cookie cutters.
7. Lift them onto greased baking sheet using broad spatula.
8. Bake in oven for about 12 minutes or until cookie springs back lightly at canter. Don't overcook them.
9. Remove them from baking sheets; cool them on wire rack.

11) Gluten-Free Cinnamon-Flavoured Flax-Cranberry Muffins

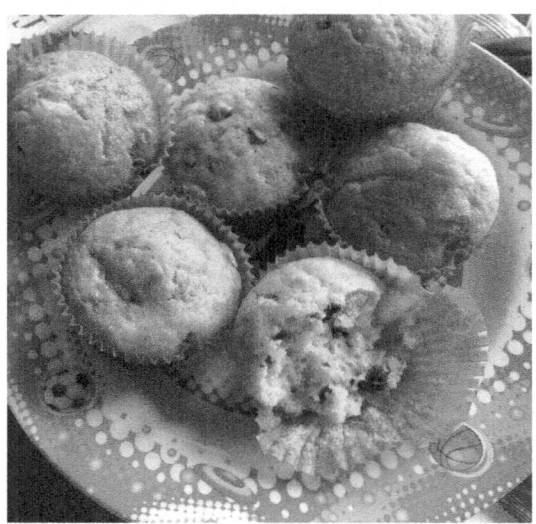

Cooking Time: 18 minutes

Yields: 12 muffins

Ingredients:

- 1 cup of flaxseed meal
- ¼ cup rice/arrowroot flour mix (or any other BTD-compliant flour)
- 3 tbsp of cinnamon
- 1 tsp of allspice
- ¼ tsp of baking soda
- ½ tsp of sea salt
- 1 tsp of lemon juice
- ¼ cup of olive oil
- 4 large eggs, beaten
- 1 tbsp of vanilla extract
- 1 cup of cranberries (optional: currants)
- ⅓ cup of agave nectar
- ¾ cup of walnuts or pecans, chopped (optional)

Directions:

1. Preheat the oven at 350°F.
2. Grease the muffin tins liberally.
3. Mix all the dry Ingredients in a bowl.
4. Mix all the wet Ingredients in a separate bowl.
5. Mix dry Ingredients with wet.
6. Let them stand for about 10 minutes for thickening.
7. Fold in cranberries.

8. Fill every muffin cup up to half way, and sprinkle them with chopped walnuts.
9. Bake them for about 15–18 minutes or until toothpick inserted at center withdraws cleanly.

12) Gluten-Free Ginger Cinnamon Cookies

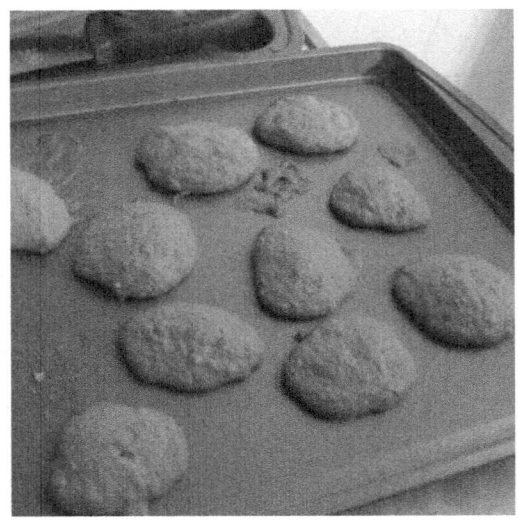

(Sorry for the mess lol)

Cooking Time: 15 minutes

Yields: 24 cookies

Ingredients:

- ➤ 2 tsp of ghee for greasing the cookie sheet
- ➤ 1½ cups of brown rice flour
- ➤ 1 tsp of ground cinnamon (or BTD-compliant spices like clove)
- ➤ 1 tsp of ginger root (powdered)
- ➤ ¼ tsp of sea salt
- ➤ 3 tbsp of molasses
- ➤ ½ cup of honey (or BTD-compliant sweetener like agave nectar)

Directions:

1. Preheat the oven at 350° F.
2. Grease the baking sheet using ghee and keep aside.
3. In a mixing bowl, combine flour, salt, and spices together.
4. Add molasses and sweetener; stir together. Shape the dough into a ball.
5. Wet your hands and take small sections; roll them into ¾-inch balls.
6. Place them 3 inches apart on the greased baking sheet.
7. Press each ball flat (¼-inch thick) using bottom of wet glass.
8. Bake them for about 12–15 minutes, until slightly brown.
9. Remove them from baking sheet immediately.

13) Nut and Honey Almond Slices

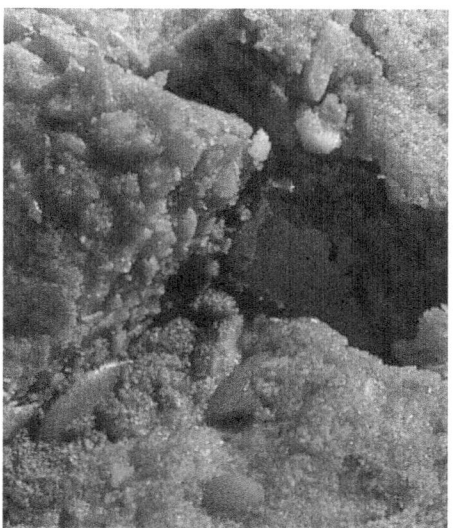

Cooking Time: 25 minutes

Servings: 3-4

Ingredients:

- 120 g (1 cup) of dates, chopped (or figs)
- 90 g (1 cup) of pecans, chopped
- 90 g (1 cup) of almonds, chopped
- 90 g (¼ cup) of honey (or agave)
- 2 eggs
- ½ cup of amaranth
- ½ cup of almond meal

Directions:

1. Preheat the oven to 350° F.
2. Beat honey and eggs together.
3. Add chopped nuts, dates, amaranth, and almond meal and mix well.
4. Place into tin lined with parchment paper and press it down well.
5. Bake in oven for about 25 minutes until brown on the top.
6. Cool it in the tin and cut it into squares.

14) Banana Oat and Buckwheat Bread

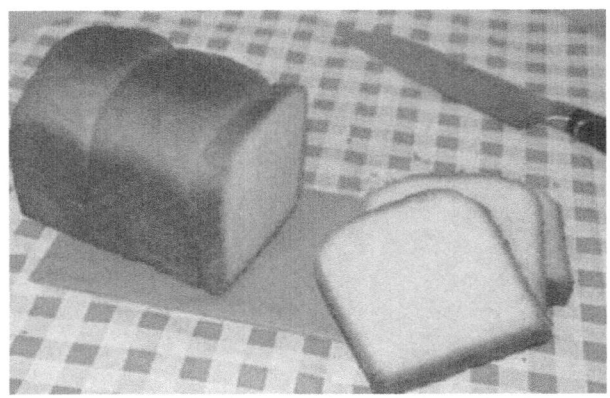

Cooking Time: 60 minutes

Yields: 1 loaf

Ingredients:

- ¾ cup of sugar (or BTD-compliant sweetener)
- ¼ cup of water
- 2–3 bananas
- 1 tsp of lemon juice (optional)
- 1 or 2 eggs, beaten
- 2 cups of flour
- 1 tsp of baking soda
- ¼ tsp of cinnamon, nutmeg, or cloves
- ½ tsp of sea salt
- 1 tsp of vanilla
- ½–1 cup of nuts, chopped (optional)

Directions:

1. Preheat the oven to 375° F.
2. Combine the wet Ingredients in one bowl.
3. Combine the dry Ingredients in another bowl.
4. Add wet Ingredients to the dry Ingredients; mix well.
5. Pour it into a loaf pan or into muffin tin.
6. Bake in oven for about 45–60 minutes or until a toothpick withdraws cleanly.

15) One-Bowl Cupcakes

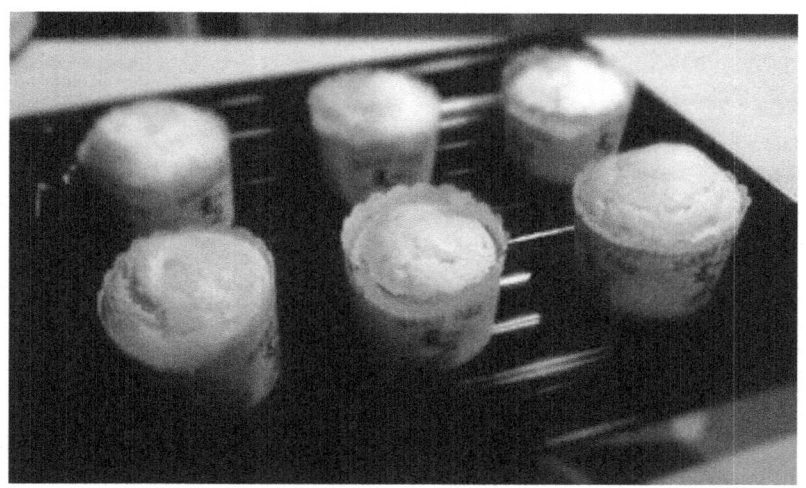

Cooking Time: 25 minutes

Yields: 12 cupcakes

Ingredients:

> - ½ cup of oil (canola or olive)
> - ½ cup of sugar (brown, white, or raw) (or ¼ cup of agave)
> - ½ of cup milk (skim, soy, 2 percent, or rice)
> - 1 cup of puree (pumpkin or banana) or 2 cups of grated zucchini plus ½ cup of cocoa
> - 1 egg
> - ½ cup of oat flour
> - 1 tsp of baking soda
> - 1½ cups of rice flour
> - ½ tsp of baking powder
> - ½ tsp of sea salt
> - ½ tsp of clove or 1 tsp of cinnamon

Directions:

1. Preheat the oven to 350° F.
2. Combine wet Ingredients.
3. On top of this mixture, sprinkle all dry Ingredients and mix until moist (don't over mix).
4. Pour batter into muffin tins using ⅓ cup and bake them for 20–25 minutes.

16) Cherry and Parsnip Bread

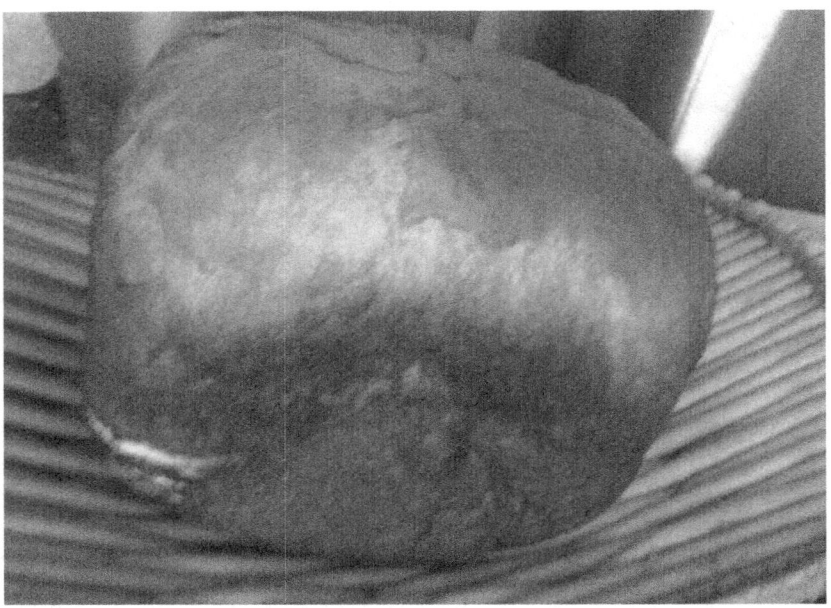

Cooking Time: 10 minutes

Yields: 1 loaf

Ingredients:

- ➢ 1 egg + 1 cup water
- ➢ 4 tsp of canola oil (or BTD-compliant substitute)
- ➢ 4 tsp of brown sugar (or BTD-compliant substitute)
- ➢ 1 tsp of sea salt
- ➢ 1 large parsnip, peeled, diced
- ➢ ⅓ cup of cherries
- ➢ 2¼ cups of whole grain spelt
- ➢ 1 pkg of dry yeast
- ➢ ⅓ cup of raisins

Directions:

1. Place all the Ingredients except raisins in a bread machine and switch it on.
2. At beep, add raisins.

17) Pineapple and Walnut Cookies

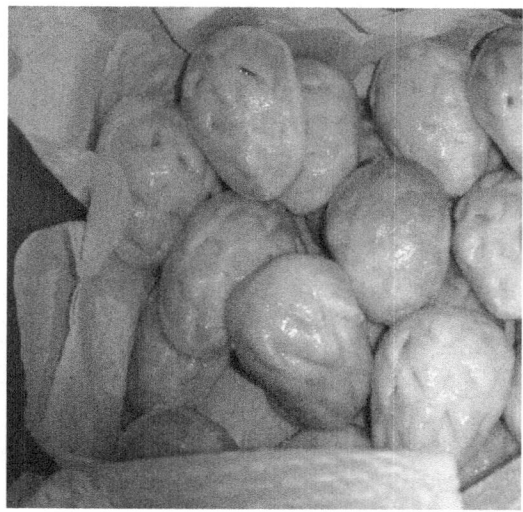

Cooking Time: 20 minutes

Yields: 12–15 cookies

Ingredients:

- ⅓ cup of brown sugar (or ¼ cup of agave)
- ⅓ cup of white sugar (or ¼ cup of agave)
- ⅓ cup of olive oil (or ghee)
- ½–¾ cup of crushed pineapple (juice drained)
- ¼ tsp of baking soda
- 1 egg
- ¼ tsp of sea salt
- 1 tsp of baking powder
- 1 tsp of vanilla (optional)
- ½ cup of walnuts, chopped
- 2 cup of spelt flour (or any BTD-compliant flour)

Directions:

1. Preheat the oven at 350° F.
2. Combine all the Ingredients together.
3. Lightly grease the cookie sheet using olive oil.
4. Drop it by spoonful onto the cookie sheet.
5. Bake them for about 15–20 minutes or until golden brown.

18) Pumpkin Vanilla–Flavoured Muffins

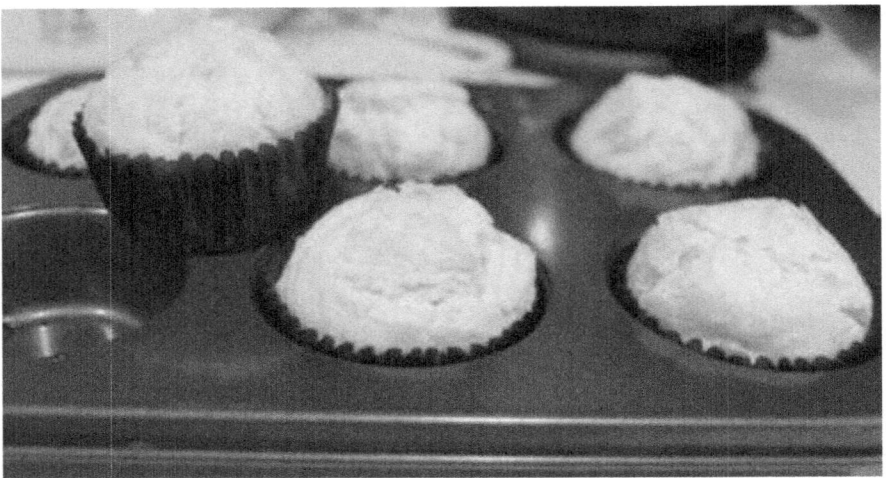

Cooking Time: 30 minutes

Yields: 6 muffins

Ingredients:

> - 3 eggs
> - 3 slices crumbled bread (Ezekiel is great)
> - 1 tsp of pumpkin spice
> - 1½ cups of pumpkin
> - 1 tsp of vanilla (optional)
> - 1 tsp of baking soda
> - 1 tsp of baking powder
> - 10 tsp of sweetener, BTD-compliant

Directions:

1. Preheat the oven to 350° F.
2. Mix all the Ingredients in the food processor; fill 6 greased muffin tins.
3. Bake them for about 25–30 minutes.
4. Let them cool and serve.

19) Fast Savoury Bread

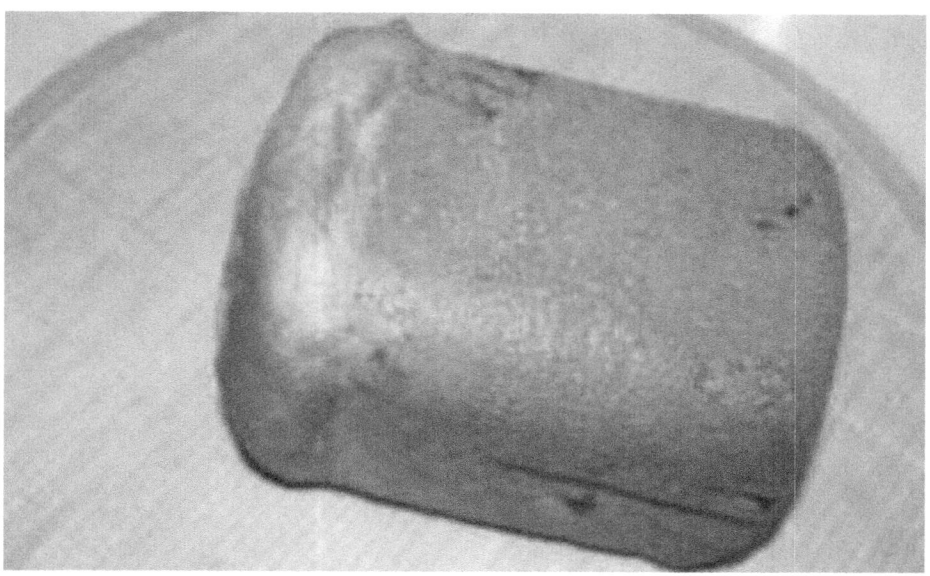

Cooking Time: 20 minutes

Yields: 1 loaf

Ingredients:

- ½ cup of brown rice flour
- 2 tsp of freshly grounded millet (optional)
- 1½ tsp of ghee
- 1 pinch of sea salt
- 1 small egg
- 1/8 tsp of chili powder (or any dry herb/spice)
- Pineapple juice or any compliant juice

Directions:

1. Whisk the egg.
2. Add sea salt and ghee and whisk once again.
3. Blend in spice and flours.
4. Mix them well by adding pineapple juice until a creamy batter is achieved.
5. Leave the mixture to soak for about 10 minutes
6. Spread it on the parchment paper
7. Bake at 350° F for about 20 minutes.

38305902R00051

Made in the USA
Middletown, DE
07 March 2019